East West RX

Wisdom of the Body Handbook

How To Combine Eastern and Western Nutrition For Optimal Balance

Susan Friedrich

1

Library of Congress Control Number: 2011904737

ISBN 978-0-9834730-0-8

EastWestRX@gmail.com

Front Cover Image: Filomena Scalise / FreeDigitalPhotos.net
Back Cover Image: Judy Slionys-Adams / Donation

I dedicate this book to

Christian, Diego, and Daniela.

PREFACE

Our bodies were bioengineered thousands of years ago before chemicals were in our environment and food. Our bodies, still today, react better using natural herbs and vitamins to achieve balance for optimal health.

It is essential that we learn to listen to our bodies. From the day we are born until the day that we die, we are in constant change. Medications, herbs, vitamins and food that were good for you yesterday, may not work for your body today. By listening to our bodies and keeping in balance, we can stay disease free, and have good energy throughout each day.

This handbook has been written for your use on how to combine Eastern and Western nutrition for a long and healthy life. Enjoy.

WISDOM OF THE BODY HANDBOOK

"The doctor ignorant of behavior and diet is like a king whose kingdom has become the enemy: the disorder grows in strength, while the body's constituents grow weak."

Mirror of Beryl – Introduction to Tibetan Medicine

There is a Spiritual and Medical Renaissance emerging as we move into the era of health practice. Instead of disease management, I want to teach people to read their own body's signals to achieve balance for excellent health. When a person becomes ill, their body's balance is lost. It takes work to get back into balance, and there is no lazy way out. As we age, it is like taking care of an antique car, we need more maintenance and TLC. We can learn to take care of ourselves at any age – from very young children to the elderly – it is never too late to learn how to read our body and get back to excellent health and balance.

In my practice I try to teach my patients how to read their body's signals to help them keep a healthy balance. I started off by making handouts for my patients, and that has turned out to be my book. After many, many years of adhering to a western diet and nutritional regimen, I now use a combination of eastern and western nutrition, herbs, vitamins, and healing techniques. I also take into consideration the food options we have, our eating habits, and then try to retrain my patients to pay attention to their own body's signals and then eat, nourish and exercise to heal themselves.

The body's chemistry is constantly changing on a daily and hourly basis. There is no set prescription for healing, and keeping our body in balance. Instead we have to learn to read the signals our body gives us and go from there. This is essential in keeping our body's immune system strong – the ability to absorb nutrients and utilize oxygen is critical to the immune function.

Usually when a patient comes to me he or she is in crises of some sort. While they are in treatment, I teach them to read their tongues in the morning and an hour after they eat to see what their body is telling them. I also ask my patients to carry around pH strips at the beginning to test themselves in the morning and an hour after eating – this will help them to understand what their body is saying, and if the body is able to absorb the nutrients being put into them. Using these simple biofeedback techniques, it is easy to learn what their body is telling them. It will help them to understand and to make intelligent choices. By using these intelligent choices, it will be easier to keep our body in balance so that it can function at an optimum level.

Oh, by the way, DO NOT EVER BRUSH YOUR TONGUE. The tongue is evidence of where you are at this time – it is a very important diagnostic tool. If the tongue is shiny as glass, or has patches of shiny with curdles and whey, or it has lumps and bumps, or it is as pale as vanilla ice cream or as purple as cabbage or as red as a Santa's suit – it is all evidence of where your body is at that very moment. It is a very important diagnostic tool for you to know what to eat and do that day to put your body in balance. More about tongues later.

Hopefully by the end of this handbook you will have the tools to bring about balance in your life. You will feel better, have more energy, and be more emotionally stable and grounded and ready to handle life's challenges.

I believe that with the tools I am giving you, you can make intelligent choices for your own health. By the way, none of us are perfect. If we overeat during the holidays, these same tools will help you to get out of crises and back on the road to good health.

First, if you are in a health crisis, you more than likely did not get there overnight unless you were in an accident, so getting back to good health will take time and you have to do your homework.   I give all of my patients homework and it is up to them to get back on the road to health and to follow through.

By using my methods, you can rebalance your body quickly once it has a problem.   Here are warning signs of our body saying "help – I am out of balance".

- Pain, body aches, cramps, restless leg
- Irregular bowel movements – normal is 2 to 3 times a day.
- Irregular menses – either too much or too little.
- Cramps related to menses.
- Bleeding for no reason
- Indigestion, gas, bloating, burping
- Sudden weight gain or weight loss
- Swelling anywhere
- Bad breath, teeth and gum problems
- Problems with your eyes
- Low energy at any time of the day
- Frequent urination or low flow urination or bedwetting
- Eye problems
- Impotence
- Infertility
- Headaches, migraines, dizziness, vertigo
- Loss of hearing, tinnitus

- Sleep problems – either getting to sleep or staying asleep.

There are many more warning signs – the above list contains just a few symptoms that many people think are normal.

Some people do not know what normal is, so here is a very short list.

- The body should be pain free – if there is pain, it is the body's way of telling you something is wrong.
- Bowel movements should be 2 to 3 times a day, no dry stools, and stools should be long and continuous. Color should not be dark or have undigested food still in it.
- Menses – timing should be regular, without pain, mood swings or clotting and fertility should not be a problem.
- Energy – your energy should be high all day long without the use of caffeine or other stimulants.

EASTERN NUTRITION BASICS – IT IS ALL ABOUT BALANCE

In Western medicine we say you can live without the Spleen, but in Eastern medicine the Spleen is digestion. The stronger the Spleen is, the better we are able to digest and absorb our nutrients. The Spleen is related to our emotional state and our relationship to Earth. It is important that we balance our nutrients and emotions for the best digestion. Our body is always looking for balance. For instance, if we over use our mental abilities and work on the computer and read too much without getting outside to breathe in fresh air, and do some physical exercise, then the Spleen is out of balance, and so is our digestion and nutrient absorption. The ability of our body to absorb nutrients results in the amount of energy our body has (Qi). FOOD = BLOOD and ENERGY (Qi). The Spleen likes warm foods and does not like to be flooded with liquids while we eat. It is better to drink liquids between meals. Soups and stews are the most absorbable foods we can eat.

In the West we describe food as containing proteins, fats, minerals, vitamins, etc. These are the chemical ingredients of food BEFORE they enter the body.

In the East, we describe food as the action of the food on the body AFTER eating. It is also all about Balance of the temperature, flavors and actions on the body. When our body is out of balance, we develop a craving to correct that imbalance and that craving is a message that we have to teach ourselves to pay attention to so we can maximize our health. The information in this book will help you to understand how foods work on our bodies so that you can choose foods to include in your diet which are tailor made for your own personal energetic needs.

FOOD TEMPERATURE

The most important category of food is its temperature.   That is the measure of the effect on the body AFTER digestion – does it warm us up or cool us down?

- *COOLING FOODS –* direct energy inwards and downwards, they cool the upper and outer parts of the body first.
- *WARMING FOODS –* move energy upwards and outwards from the core and warm us from the inside out.
- *VERY HOT FOODS –* (like chili peppers) heat us up intensely and then cool us down quickly by sweating out the hot.

Warmer foods speed us up!!!
Cooler foods slow us down.

Hint: If you want to speed up your metabolism you eat warmer foods (not cold salads)!!

Here are some very general guidelines for knowing if a food is warming or cooling:

- Plants which take longer to grow (like root vegetables, ginger, carrots, rutabaga, parsnips, and cabbage) tend to be warmer than fast growing foods like lettuce, squash, radish and cucumbers.
- Foods with high water content tend to be more cooling (like melons, cucumber, and lettuce).
- Dried foods tend to be warmer than their fresh counterparts.
- Raw food is more cooling than cooked food. Food eaten cold is more cooling.
- Foods with blue, green or purple colors are more cooling than red, orange, or yellow foods (a green apple is more cooling than a red one).
- Chemically fertilized foods which are forced to grow quickly tend to be cooler (this includes most commercially grown fruits and vegetables), than the same food grown naturally.
- Some chemicals that are added to foods may produce heat reactions within the body.
- The finer we cut our food, the more heat it releases to our bodies and raises blood sugar levels, which in turn affects our thought patterns.

- Chewing food more thoroughly creates warmth – it even warms up cooling foods and improves digestion.
- Moderately cooked food supports a more refined consciousness.

The temperature of the food also depends on how it is prepared and cooked. Cooking methods that involve more cooking time, higher temperatures, greater pressure, dryness and/or air circulation cause foods to be more warming.

Microwave cooking alters food enough to cause, upon ingestion, structural, functional and immunological changes in the body – they transform the amino acid L-proline into D-proline which is a proven toxin to the nervous system, liver and kidneys.

- *RAW* foods are more cooling
- *STEAMED* foods are cooling or neutral
- *BOILED* foods are neutral
- *STEWED, STIR FRIED and BAKED* foods are more warming.
- *DEEP FRIED, ROASTED, GRILLED and BBQ* foods are more heating.

Longer and Slower methods of cooking will produce more warming effects than quicker methods.

FOODS THAT REMOVE HEAT
AND COOL THE BODY

Asparagus
Banana
Elderflower
Lettuce
Beansprouts
Salt
Wheat
All Citrus Fruits
Radish
Celery
Eggplant
Bok Choy
Zucchini
Tempeh
Saffron
Yogurt
Spearmint
White Peppercorn
Mulberry
Sage
Loquat
Chicory
Dill
Licorice
Kelp and all
Seaweeds

Aubergine
Chicken Eggs
Grapefruit
Millet
Peppermint
Tofu
Apples
Persimmons
Tomato
Mushrooms
Spinach
Broccoli
Soy Milk
Barley
Greens
Crab
Nettles
Cilantro
Strawberry
Chamomile
Mandarin Orange
Coriander
Fennel
Pomegranate
Dandelion Greens
and Root

Bamboo Shoots
Clams
Lemon
Mung Bean
Potato
Watermelon
Pears
Cantalope
Cucumber
Swiss Chard
Cabbage
Caulifower
Sprouts
Quinoa
Kudzu
Clams
Red Clover
Marjoram
Black Sesame Seeds
Apple
Mango
Cumin
Lemongrass

FOODS TO DRIVE OUT THE COLD

Amasake	Anchovy	Basil
Bay Leaf	Black Pepper	Brown Sugar
Butter	Capers	Cayenne
Cherry	Chestnuts	Chicken
Chive Seeds	Coconut Milk	Coriander Seed
Dill Seed	Fennel Seed	Garlic
Ginger	Kohlrabi	Lamb
Leek	Lychee	Longan
Malt Sugar	Mussels	Mustard
Nutmeg	Onion	Peach
Pine Nuts	Rosemary	Scallion
Shrimp	Soy	Spearmint
Squash	Sweet Potato	Rice
Trout	Turnip	Vinegar
Walnuts	Wine	Cinnamon
Green Pepper	Red Pepper	Soybean Oil
Carp	Brown Sugar	Dates
Clove	Eel	Guava
Ham	Kumquat	Nutmeg
Peach	Raspberry	Sunflower Seeds
Sweet Basil	Allspice	Anise
Caraway	Cardamom	Cloves
Fenugreek	Hawthorne Berries	Kelp
Marjoram	Mustard	Orange Peel
Oregano	Paprika	Parsley
Rosemary	Sage	Sesame Seeds

FOODS THAT RESOLVE DAMPNESS

Aduki beans
Barley
Corn
Green Tea
Job's Tears
Lemon
Mushrooms
Parsley
Radish
Turnip
Asparagus

Alfalfa
Buckwheat tea
Daikon
Horseradish
Kidney Beans
Mackerel
Mustard Leaf
Pumpkin
Rye
Umeboshi Plum

Anchovy
Celery
Garlic
Jasmine Tea
Kohlrabi
Marjoram
Onion
Quinoa
Scallion
White Fungus

BODY RHYTHMS – CIRCADIAN RHYTHMS

Our bodies wake up and slow down according to the sunrise and sundown times. Since your metabolism peaks at about noon, it is better for your body to have a larger breakfast and lunch and smaller dinner. By eating this way our body can have time to digest what we have eaten. Our body starts to slow down to get ready for a good night's sleep after 6:00 p.m. and reenergize. It is best to not eat after 6:00 p.m.

Since our central nervous system has to reboot at night, it needs total darkness. That means that we need to turn off the television and computer in the room that we sleep in. If we have to recharge our cell phones, it is better to do that in another room also. Never sleep in a room with a television or computer turned on. Light and sound act as activators to our nervous system.

FOOD FLAVORS

There are five main flavors that are related to the organs. The flavors have to be balanced. If a flavor is generally helpful for an organ function, too much of that flavor has an opposite and weakening effect. When we talk about flavors, it means the natural flavor of a food. Remember that the body always looks for balance and too much of any flavor can throw us off our natural balance. The body needs a little bit of all flavors to stay balanced and a variety of many foods.

SALTY FLAVOR enters the Kidneys and Bladder and moves inward and downward going towards the center and root of the body. It also moistens, softens and detoxifies going into the muscles and glands, and regulating the moisture balance in the body. Salty moistens dryness and softens hardened lymph nodes and cataracts as well as relaxes the knotted and stiff muscles and glands; improves digestion and detoxifies the body, and can purge the bowels. Salt counteracts toxins in the body. Salt has a cooling nature and attunes the body during the cold season. Salty foods moisten and calm the thin, dry, nervous person, but should not be used as much by a damp, overweight, lethargic person. Seaweeds have no restrictions because their iodine and trace minerals speed up the metabolism and detoxify. Any salt used as seasoning should be natural unprocessed sea salt. Excess saltiness is counteracted by the addition of sweet foods.

A little saltiness supplements the quality of the Blood, but in Excess it can congeal the Blood and stress the Heart. Excess saltiness is associated with deficient muscles and flesh with a lack of strength in the large bones and depression. Remember the body looks for BALANCE.

FOODS THAT ARE SALTY

Seaweeds	Kelp	Kombu
Dulse	Barley	Millet
Miso	Pickles	Umeboshi Plum
Sesame Salt	Salt	

SOUR FLAVOR enters the Liver and Gall Bladder and causes an astringent effect – they stimulate contraction and absorption. Sour is associated with the Wood element. A diet that has an excess of sour is associated with weakening of the Spleen, overproduction of saliva by the Liver and injury to the muscles. You can use Sour flavors for leaking and sagging conditions that involve loss of body fluids like sweating and diarrhea, hemorrhoids and uterine prolapse – it dries up and firms up tissues. Sour also counteracts the affects of fatty foods, benefits digestion and prevents stagnation. They also stimulate secretions from the gall bladder and pancreas and usually lower the acidity level in the intestines. Sour is also a blood activator and stagnation eliminator. Sour flavors lower blood sugar (lemons and grapefruit). Sour is most active in the Liver where it counteracts the effects of greasy food, breaking down fats and protein – it also helps to dissolve minerals, improves stimulation and strengthens the Lungs. Sour organizes the scattered mental patterns. Tendons and Ligaments do not like a lot of sour food. Too much sour flavors can be counteracted by pungent foods.

A little Sour flavor will help to cleanse, detoxify and tone our systems, however in excess they can cause over-contraction and over retention of moisture and can injure the muscles. Remember the body looks for BALANCE.

FOODS THAT ARE SOUR

Lemons
Blackberry Leaves
Pickles
Sour Apple (crab apple)

Grapefruit
Hawthorne Berry
Rose Hip

Sour Plum

Black and Green Tea
Lime
Saurkraut

SOUR AND BITTER

Vinegar

SOUR AND PUNGENT

Leek

SOUR AND SWEET

Aduki Bean
Cheese
Mango
Sourdough Bread
Yogurt

Apple
Grape
Olive
Tangerine

Blackberry
Huckleberry
Raspberry
Tomato

BITTER FLAVOR enters the Heart, Small Intestine and Upper Respiratory System, draining and drying as it goes downwards in the body. Bitter is associated with the Fire element. A diet that has an excess of bitter is associated with Spleen energy, dryness and congestion of the Stomach energy and a withering of the skin. Bitter is used to draw out dampness and heat, improves appetite, contracts, lowers fever, dries fluids, induces bowel movements and stimulates digestion. Bitter reduces the excess person and is helpful for inflammations, infections and constipation. It clears heat and cleans arteries of damp mucus deposits of cholesterol and fats and tends to lower blood pressure. Bitter foods also drains damp associated with Candida yeast, parasites, swellings, skin eruptions, abscesses, tumors, cysts, obesity and edema. People who are slow, overweight and lethargic can most benefit from bitter flavors. People who are cold, weak, thin, nervous, dry and have bone diseases should limit bitter in their diet. Bitter can be counteracted by Salty foods.

A little Bitter flavor will draw out dampness; however in excess it can deplete the QI and moisture in the body, dry up the energy in the Spleen and congest the Stomach. Remember the body looks for BALANCE.

FOODS THAT ARE BITTER

Celery

Burdock

Pau d'Arco

Alfalfa

Rye

Dandelion Leaf

Chamomile

Chaparral

Bitter Melon

Green Tea

Yarrow

Hops

Echinacea

Romaine Lettuce

Dark Chocolate

BITTER AND PUNGENT

Citrus peel

Turnip

Radish

White Pepper

Scallion

BITTER AND SWEET

Quinoa

Celery

Amaranth

Lettuce

Asparagus

Papaya

BITTER AND SOUR

Vinegar

SWEET FLAVOR enters the Spleen, Pancreas and Stomach. Sweet flavors moisten the body, nourishes us and mildly stimulates circulation. The Earth element is associated with Sweet flavors. Sweet is harmonizing and retarding. Sweet flavors also removes cold, lubricates dryness in the mouth, throat and lungs. Sweet flavors should be accompanied by small amounts of Bitter, Salty, Pungent and Sour foods. Fruits are more cleansing and cooling. Sweet flavors in warming foods send energy upward and outward and harmonizes the body, slowing it and relaxing it. Sweet foods build the yin of the body – the tissues and fluids – they strengthen weakness and deficiency in general. Complex carbohydrates such as grains and vegetables are good for a cold or deficient person. Sweet is good for the Liver and soothes aggressive Liver emotions such as anger. The dry, cold, nervous, thin, weak or scattered person needs sweet flavors. A sluggish, overweight person with mucus should take very little sweet flavors. A diet with excess sweet is associated with achy bones, unbalanced Kidneys, full Heart energy and hair loss. Sweet can be counteracted by the addition of Sour foods.

A little Sweet flavor will harmonize with other flavors to moisten us, but in excess Sweet will form Phlegm and Heat causing Damp conditions. Too much Sweet retards calcium metabolism and initiates skeletal problems like bone loss and arthritis. Too much also makes our blood acidic, which makes our hair fall out, destroys B Vitamins and depletes the body of minerals. Remember the body looks for BALANCE.

FOODS THAT ARE SWEET

Most Carbohydrates	Grains	Vegetables
Nuts	Seeds	Fruit
Rice	Spearmint	Sweet Potato
Mochi	Amasake	Molasses
Sunflower Seeds	Pinenuts	Walnut
Cherry	Cabbage	Carrot
Shiitake Mushrooms	Figs	Yam
Peas	Apple	Apricot
Dates	Grapes	Grapefruit
Olives	Papaya	Peach
Pear	Strawberry	Tomato
Beets	Celery	Chard
Eggplant	Kuzu	Lettuce
Potato	Squash	Almond
Chestnut	Coconut	Sesame Seeds
Barley	Raw Honey	Sugar
Milk	Pasta	Ice Cream
White Sugar		

SWEET AND SALTY

Duck	Pork	Watermelon

SWEET AND WARM

Chicken	Lamb

PUNGENT FLAVOR enters the Lungs and Large Intestine, disperses stagnation and breaks through Mucus conditions such as the common cold. Pungent flavor also improves digestion, which is ruled by the Spleen and Pancreas and expels gas from the intestines. The Metal element is associated with Hot, Pungent and Aromatic flavors. The use of pungents needs to be combined with a tonifying diet. When a pungent flavor has a warming energy, it stimulates circulation of energy and blood, moving the energy upwards and outwards. Pungents stimulate blood circulation and improves a sluggish liver function. People who are sluggish, heavy or have damp and mucus conditions are benefited by pungent flavors. With Qi Stagnation problems avoid too much pungent. Pungency is diminished by cooking. Raw honey has a pungent, drying effect on the body after digestion – it dries up damp, overweight and mucus conditions. Pungent can be counteracted by the addition of bitter foods. A diet that has an excess of pungent is associated with muscle knots, slack pulse, a damaged Shen, and unhealthy fingernails and toenails. Excess pungent flavors over stimulate and exhaust the Qi and blood. This can be counteracted by the addition of bitter foods.

A little Pungent flavor is good to break through mucus, but too much will over stimulate and exhaust the QI and Blood, cause muscle knots, slack pulse and damage the Shen, and will cause unhealthy finger nails and toe nails. Remember the body looks for BALANCE.

FOODS THAT ARE PUNGENT FLAVOR

Mint	Ginger	Cayenne
Elder Flower	Scallion	Garlic
Chamomile	Mugwort	Black Pepper
Hot Green and Red Peppers	Cinnamon	Fennel
Dill	Caraway	Anise
Coriander	Cumin	Onion
Horseradish	Spearmint	Rosemary
Cloves	Basil	Nutmeg
Marjoram	Radish	Taro
Turnip	Kohlrabi	Cabbage
Chile Pepper	Yogurt	

FOOD MOVEMENTS

As you know we should eat a balanced diet using various flavors, temperatures, etc. We also need to balance our diets as to how the food moves in our body. Foods also move in different directions in the body.

Foods that move from the INSIDE towards the OUTSIDE induce perspiration and reduce fever. Inward symptoms such as constipation and abdominal swelling, should be treated by outward moving foods in combination with other foods that cleanse the internal regions of the body. Foods prepared with Ginger tend to move outward. Generally, foods that are warm and hot and have a pungent and sweet flavor tend to move UPWARDS or OUTWARDS.

Foods that move from the OUTSIDE towards the INSIDE ease bowel movements and abdominal swelling. Generally, foods that are cold that have a sour, salty or bitter flavor tend to move DOWNARDS and INWARDS.

Foods that move UPWARD towards the upper region of the body relieve diarrhea, prolapse of the anus and uterus and of a falling stomach. In general, leaves and flowers move upwards. Foods prepared with wine tend to move upward.

Foods that move DOWN towards the lower region of the body can relieve vomiting, hiccupping and asthma. In general, roots, seeds and fruits move downwards. You can treat symptoms such as vomiting, hiccupping, coughing, etc with foods that move downwards. Foods prepared with salt tend to move downwards.

Some foods move in two directions.

Glossy foods, such as honey and spinach facilitate movements. Glossy foods are good for constipation and internal dryness.

Obstructive foods such as guava and olives obstruct movement. Obstructive foods are good for diarrhea and seminal emissions. Outward symptoms such as excessive perspiration, premature ejaculation, seminal emission, and frequent urination should be treated by foods that can obstruct. Foods prepared with vinegar tend to become obstructive.

FOODS THAT MOVE UPWARD
Pungent, Sweet, Bitter

Abalone	Apricot	Beef
Beets	Black Fungus	Black Sesame
Black Soybean	Cabbage	Carp
Carrot	Celery	Cherry
Eggs	Chicken	Corn Silk
	Dry Mandarin	
Crab Apple	Orange Peel	Duck
Eel	Fig	Grape
Guava Leaf	Raw Honey	Kidney Bean
Kohlrabi	Licorice	Lotus Fruit
Raw Milk	Olive	Oyster
Peanuts	Pineapple	Plum
Pork	Potato	
Pumpkin	Radish Leaf	Red Beans
Adzuki Beans	Saffron	Shiitake Mushrooms
String Beans	Sunflower Seeds	Sweet Rice
Sweet Potato	Taro	Sugar
Yellow Soybean		

FOODS THAT MOVE OUTWARD
Pungent, Sweet

Black Pepper	Cinnamon	Cottonseed
Ginger	Green Pepper	Red Pepper
Soybean Oil	White Pepper	

FOODS THAT MOVE DOWNWARD
Cold, Warm, Sweet, Sour

Apple	Bamboo Shoots	Banana
Barley	Bean Curd	Egg
Clam - Freshwater	Button Mushroom	Cucumber
Eggplant	Grapefruit	Hawthorn fruit
Kumquat	Job's Ears	Lettuce
Litchi	Loquat	Mango
Mung Beans	Muskmelon	Peach
Persimmon	Spinach	Star Fruit - Carambola
Strawberry	Sugar Cane Juice	Tangerine
Water Chestnut	Watermelon	Wheat
Wheat Bran		

FOODS THAT MOVE INWARD
Cold, Bitter, Salty

Clams	Crab	Hops
Kelp	Lettuce	Sea Salt
Sea Grass	Seaweed	

EASTERN NUTRITION
BASIC TERMINOLOGY

YIN – The Yin is the water in the body (lymphatics). When we have problems with our Yin, it has been happening for a long time. We need Time to replenish – rest is vital – we need to avoid stimulating foods which use up our energy – avoid coffee, alcohol, sugar, heating and pungent flavors. Depleted Yin needs sea food, seaweed, meats, nuts, seeds, beans and MOIST, COOLING foods. A small amount of dairy is good, but not too much as to cause dampness. To tonify Yin use sweet, sour and salty flavors along with very small amounts of bitter and pungent.

FOODS THAT TONIFY THE YIN

Apples	Asparagus	Cheese
Eggs	Clams	Crabs
Duck	Honey	Kidney Beans
Lemons	Mango	Milk
Oysters	Peas	Pears
Pineapples	Pomegranate	Pork
Rabbit	String beans	Tofu
Tomato	Watermelon	Yams
Seaweeds	Algae	Kelp

YANG- The Yang is the fire of the body – it keeps us warm and provides heat for all the body functions. If the Yang cools down too much, our metabolism slows down, and becomes sluggish, cold and we lose the joy of life. In order to keep the Yang warm, we need to do physical exercise and actively participate in life in order to produce yang. We need to cook our foods longer so that they penetrate the body deeper. Do not use very hot foods, as it will heat up the body and then cool it down by sweating. It is better to eat sweet, pungent and warming foods.

FOODS THAT WARM THE YANG

Basil	Chestnuts	Chive seed
Cinnamon	Cloves	Dill
Fennel	Fenugreek	Garlic
Ginger	Lamb	Lobster
Nutmeg	Pistachio	Raspberry
Rosemary	Sage	Shrimp
Anise	Thyme	Walnuts
Cardomon	Trout	

QI - To make QI (our body's natural energy), we combine Food and Air by breathing, physical exercise and postural alignment. Qi can become stagnant by tension and a sedentary lifestyle. To support and increase our QI, we need complex carbohydrates along with fresh and organic vegetables. Irradiation and microwave cooking depletes the level of QI in our food. The cause of Qi Stagnation can also be emotional. To get the Qi moving again, we need to combine pungent foods and then take into account whether the stagnation has caused either Heat, Cold or Deficiency.

FOODS THAT MOVE THE QI

Beef
Coconuts
Figs
Grapes
Lentils
Mackerel
Oats
Rabbit
Sweet Potato
Sturgeon
Basil
Carrots
Cloves
Garlic
Orange Peel
Tangerine Peel
Ginger

Cherry
Dates
Ginseng
Ham
Licorice
Algae
Octopus
Brown Rice
Mushrooms
Tofu
Caraway
Cayenne
Coriander
Marjoram
Radish
Turmeric
Fennel

Chicken
Eel
Goose
Herring
Longan
Molasses
Potato
Royal Jelly
Squash
Yam
Cardamon
Chives
Dill
Mustard
Star Anise
Black Pepper

BLOOD – the amount and quality of our blood depends on the available liquids and nourishment in our body. In other words, it depends on the strength of our Spleen. Blood also enables our thoughts and emotions to be grounded. When our Blood is undernourished we have separation of the Yin and Yang and we are not grounded. When we are not grounded, we cannot sleep. Physical activity helps to circulate the Blood, however, rest in the early afternoon helps the Liver to renew the Blood during the day. To improve Blood, eat well using a large variety of foods from all the flavors, temperatures and movements so that everything is balanced. When we have stagnant Blood, it is usually a manifestation of stagnant QI manifesting in a physical form. Foods that move Blood are warm in nature, so it is important to be cautious of signs of Heat and not over use them.

FOODS THAT MOVE BLOOD

Aduki Beans
Beets
Dandelion

Dates
Kidney Beans
Algae
Oyster
Spinach
Amasake
Chestnut
Crab
Onion
Sturgeon
Cayenne Pepper

Apricots
Bone Marrow
Dang Gui

Figs
Liver
Nettle
Parsley
Brown Rice
Aubergine
Chili Pepper
Hawthorn Berry
Peach
Vinegar
Buffalo

Beef
Eggs
Dark Leafy
Greens
Grapes
Longan
Octopus
Sardines
Watercress
Brown Sugar
Chive
Mustard
Scallion
Lotus Root

DAMPNESS– when the body cannot transform moisture in the body, it is usually a weakness of the Spleen, Kidney and Lungs. We need to avoid raw, cold, sweet or rich foods and too much fluids, especially while eating. Liquids should be ingested in between meals, not during meals. Dairy, pork, roasted nuts, juices, bread, yeast, beer, bananas, sugar, sweeteners and saturated fats contribute to dampness. These foods counteract the dampness.

FOODS THAT COUNTERACT DAMPNESS

Aduki Beans	Alfalfa	Anchovy
Barley	Buckwheat Tea	Celery
Corn	Daikon	Garlic
Green Tea	Horseradish	Jasmine Tea
Job's Tears	Kidney Beans	Kohlrabi
Lemon	Mackerel	Marjoram
Mushrooms	Mustard	Onion
Parsley	Pumpkin	Quinoa
Radish	Rye	Scallion
Turnips	Umeboshi Plums	White Fungus
Cabbage		

COLD – Cold can penetrate the body in various ways – as a pathogen such as a virus, from a deficiency of the Yang, with overconsumption of cold foods and liquids, and with emotional fear. Cold causes contractions of the muscles, joints and organs and obstructs the flow of energy (QI) and blood. For all levels of cold we use the warming methods of preparing food. For chronic cold conditions, we use warm and sweet foods. For acute cold conditions we use warm and pungent foods to drive the cold to the surface of the body and cause sweating to release the cold.

FOODS THAT RELEASE COLD

Amasake
Bay Leaf
Butter
Cherries
Chives
Dill
Ginger
Leek
Malt Sugar
Nutmeg
Pine Nuts
Shrimp
Squash
Turnip
Wine

Anchovy
Black Pepper
Capers
Chestnuts
Coconut Milk
Fennel
Kohlrabi
Lychee
Mussels
Onion
Rosemary
Soy
Sweet Potato
Vinegar

Basil
Brown Sugar
Cayenne
Chicken
Coriander
Garlic
Lamb
Longan
Mustard
Peach
Scallion
Spearmint
Trout
Walnut

HEAT – There are two types of HEAT. FALSE HEAT is when we deplete our Yin which cools and lubricates us and can no longer keep us cool. TRUE HEAT enters our body in various ways – as a hot pathogen that penetrates our defenses and causes inflammation and irritation, as overconsumption of heating foods, as over strain of our body which heats up all our systems, as over exposure to a hot environment, and on an emotional level, by not resolving our problems and not expressing our emotions, which causes stagnation and dampness.

FOODS THAT REDUCE HEAT

Asparagus	Aubergine	Bamboo Shoots
Banana	Chicken Egg Whites	Clams
Elderflower	Grapefruit	Lemons
Lettuce	Millet	Mung Beans
Bean Sprouts	Peppermint	Potato
Salt	Tofu	Watermelon
Wheat		

50

FOODS THAT CAUSE PHLEGM

All Dairy - milk   All Carbs   Pasta

FOODS THAT RESOLVE PHLEGM

Almond	Apple Peel	Clam
Daikon	Garlic	Grapefruit
Lemon Peel	Licorice	Marjoram
Mushroom	Mustard	Olive
Onion	Orange Peel	Pear
Pepper	Peppermint	Persimmon
Plantain	Radish	Seaweed
Shiitake		
Mushroom	Shrimp	Tangerine Peel
Black and Green		
Tea	Thyme	Walnut
Watercress	Mandarin Orange	Mustard Greens
Carrot	Pumpkin	Celery
Salt Water Clam		

FOODS THAT DRAIN WATER

Aduki Bean	Alfalfa	Anchovy
Barley	Black Soybean	Broad Bean
Celery	Clams	Fenugreek
Frogs	Grape	Job's Tears
Kelp	Lettuce	Mackerel
Sardine	Seaweed	

FOODS THAT LOWER BLOOD SUGAR

Grapefruit
Goat Milk and
Yogurt
Licorice
Flax Seed
Millet
Mung Beans
Radish
Asparagus
Avocado
Blueberry

Abalone
Goose

Lemons

Clams and Broth
Green Tea
Wheat Grass
Brown Rice
Garbanzo Beans
Artichoke
Yam
Pear
Huckleberry
Raw Cow's Milk
and Yogurt
Beef

Sour Flavors

Stevia
Greens
Quinoa
Oats
String Beans
Turnip
Spinach
Plum
Dandelion Root

Chicken
Fish

FOODS THAT DESTROY OR EXPEL PARASITES

Mint
Scallion
Mugwort

Cayenne
Garlic

Elderflower
Chamomile

FOODS THAT ACT ON VARIOUS ORGANS

Bladder	Cinnamon, fennel, grapefruit peel, watermelon
Gallbladder	Chicory, corn silk
Heart	Egg, Cinnamon, crab apple, green pepper, longan, lotus fruit, raw milk, mung bean, muskmelon, persimmon, red pepper, small red beans, adzuki beans, saffron, watermelon, wheat, wine
Kidneys	Black sesame seeds, black soybean, caraway, carp, chestnut, eggs, chives, cinnamon, freshwater clams, clove, cuttle fish, dill, duck, eel, fennel, grape, grapefruit peel, Job's tears, lotus fruit, mutton, oyster, plum, pork, salt, star anise, string bean, tangerine, walnut, wheat
Large Intestine	Bean curd, black fungus, black pepper, cabbage, carp, castor bean, corn, cucumber, eggplant, fig, honey, lettuce, nutmeg, persimmon, rice bran, salt, spinach, sweet basil, taro, white pepper, yellow soybean

Liver	Black sesame seed, brown sugar, celery, chicory, chive, freshwater clam, corn silk, crab, crab apple, cuttlefish, eel, hawthorne fruits, leek, litchi, loquat, peppermint, plum, saffron, sour plum, star anise, vinegar, wine
Lungs	Carrot, cinnamon, button mushroom, coriander, crab apple, duck, garlic, ginger, ginseng, grape, green onion, raw honey, Job's tears, mustard, leek, licorice, loquat, maltose, raw milk, olive, peanut, pear, peppermint, persimmon, radish, sugar cane, sweet basil, tangerine, walnut, water chestnut, wine
Small Intestine	Red beans, adzuki beans, salt, spinach
Spleen	Barley, bean curd, beef, black soybean, brown sugar, carp, carrot, chestnut, chicken, cinnamon, clove, coriander, cucumber, dates, dill, eel, eggplant, fig, garlic, ginger, ginseng, grape, grapefruit peel, green pepper, hawthorn fruit, raw honey, Job's tears, licorice, litchi, longan, loquat, lotus fruit, malt, mutton, nutmeg, peanuts, pork, radish leaf, red pepper, rice, squash, star anise, string bean, sweet basil, sweet rice, wheat, sugar, yellow soybean

Stomach	Barley, bean curd, beef, bitter gourd, black fungus, black pepper, brown sugar, cabbage, caraway, carp, celery, chestnut, chicken, chive, clams - saltwater and freshwater, clove, button mushroom, corn, crab, cucumber, dates, eggplant, fennel, garlic, ginger, green onion, hawthorn fruit, kelp, lettuce, licorice, raw milk, mung bean, muskmelon, olive, pear, pork, radish, radish leaf, rice bran, rice, salt, shiitake mushroom, squash, sugar cane, sweet basil, sweet rice, tangerine, taro, vinegar, water chestnut, watermelon, wheat bran, white pepper, wine

FOODS FOR SYMPTOMS

Acidosis	Greens, lemons, limes, seaweed, wheat grass, kale
Appetite - Improve it	Red and green peppers
Bleeding - will stop the bleeding	Black fungus, chestnut, chicken eggshell, cottonseed, cuttlebone, guava, spinach, vinegar
Blood coagulations - disperse them	Brown sugar, chives, crab, hawthorne fruit, vinegar
Bowel Movements - Induce them	Seaweeds, avocado, sesame oil, castor bean
Calms the Spirit	Chamomile, licorice, lily flower
Edema	Garlic,
Eliminate sputum	Saltwater clams, pears, radish, sea grass, seaweed
Headache	Sweet basil, Peppermint
Lubricate dryness	Bean curd, eggs, raw honey, raw milk, pears, pork, spinach, sugar cane juice, yellow soybean
Lubricate intestines	Banana, raw milk, peach, walnut, watermelon
Lubricate Lungs	Apple, apricot, eggs, ginseng, loquat, mandarin orange, peanuts, persimmon, strawberry, sugar

Menopause Symptoms	Cinnamon stick, black cohosh, seaweeds
Perspiration - stop it	Peach
Perspiration - induce it	Cinnamon, coriander, ginger, green onion, marjoram, rosemary
Produce fluids	Apple, apricot, bean curd, coconut, dates, ham, lemon, licorice, litchi, raw milk, peach, pear, plum, sour plum, star fruit, strawberry, sugar cane juice, tomato, sugar
Promote Blood Circulation	Black soybean, brown sugar, chestnut, eel, peach, saffron, sweet basil, wine
Promote Digestion	Apple, coriander, ginseng, green pepper, nutmeg, papaya, pineapple, plum, radish, red pepper, sweet basil, tomato
Promote Energy Circulation	Caraway, chive, dill, dry mandarin orange peel, fennel, garlic, kumquat, litchi, marjoram, radish leaf, spearmint, star anise,sweet basil, tangerine
Promote Milk Lactation	Carp, lettuce, dill seed

Promote Urination	Asparagus, barley, cabbage, carrot, coconut, coffee, corn, corn silk, cucumber, grape, Job's tears, kidney beans, lettuce, mandarin orange, mango, mung beans, muskmelon, onion, pineapple, plum, star fruit, sugar cane juice, water chestnut,watermelon
Quench Thirst	Crab apple, cucumber, loquat, mango, muskmelon, persimmon, pineapple
Reduce Fever	Muskmelon, star fruit, water chestnut
Relieve Cough	Kumquat, mandarin orange, tangerine, thyme
Relieve Diarrhea	Guava, sunflower seeds
Relieve Hot Sensation in the Body	Eggs, crab, mung bean, sea grass
Relieve Pain	Raw Honey, litchi, spearmint, squash,
Seminal Ejaculaton	Walnut, black fungus
Sharpen Vision	Abalone, bitter gourd, cucumber, freshwater clam, cuttlefish
Softens Hardness	Saltwater clam, kelp, oyster, sea grass, seaweed
Stomach Ache	Fennel seed,
Tone Up Blood Deficiency	Beef, Eggs, cuttlefish, breast milk, oyster, spinach
Tone Up Energy Deficiency	Bean curd, beef, brown sugar, chicken, eel, licorice, mutton, rice, potato, sweet potato

Tone up Heart	Wheat, coffee
Tone up Kidneys	Black sesame seed, string beans, wheat, kidneys
Tone up Liver	Black sesame seed, liver
Tone up Lungs	Job's Tears, raw milk
Tone up Spleen	Beef, carp, ham, Job's tears, rice, potato, string bean, sweet potato, yellow soybean
Tone up Stomach	Beef, raw milk, rosemary
Toxins - Counteract	Abalone, banana, bean curd, black soybean, castor bean, egg whites, freshwater clams, cucumber, dates, fig, raw honey, Job's tears, soklrabi, radish, salt, sesame oil, red beans, star fruit, vinegar
Urination - stops leakage	Raspberry
Vomiting	Star anise, fennel seed, clove, ginger,

COOKING OILS

There is a lot of confusion regarding which cooking oils to use. The healthiest and best product to use for cooking is either butter or ghee, which is clarified butter. The best oil to use in room temperature or for cold food is cold pressed extra virgin olive oil.

Saturated fatty acids are the most stable when exposed to heat and light, and have the fewest rancidity problems, which maintain their integrity for cooking. Oils that have a high percentage of saturated fatty acids are your next best choice for cooking. Saturated fats are solid at room temperature.

Monounsaturated fatty acids are moderately stable, but not as good as butter, ghee or saturated fatty acids when exposed to heat. Monounsaturated oils are liquid at room temperature, but solid in the refrigerator.

Polyunsaturated fatty acids are unstable and tend to produce significant amounts of free radicals when exposed to heat. These oils **should never be used for cooking.** Polyunsaturated fats are liquid at room temperature and in the refrigerator. Polyunsaturated oils, margarines and shortening cause a greater risk of heart attack, cancer and elevated cholesterol. Both heat and air speed up the deterioration of oils. Keep them in closed containers in a dark area where the temperature does not exceed 65 degrees F. The effect of light on unsaturated fatty acids is worse than air, and turns the oils into free radical chains.

COOKING OILS				
	%Saturated Fats	%Monounsaturated Fats	%Polyunsaturated Fats	
Avocado Oil	12.1%	73.8%	14.1%	
Butter / Ghee	65.0%	5.0%	2.0%	This is the best choice for cooking as it can stand up to heat
Canola Oil	7.4%	61.6%	31.0%	
Coconut Oil	91.9%	6.2%	1.9%	Coconut oil is one of the best to cook with after butter and ghee, as it can stand up to heat.

Cold Pressed Extra Virgin Olive Oil	13.8%	75.9%	10.3%	Cold pressed extra virgin olive oil should never be used for cooking as it turns into a transfat under low heat or light exposure. It is best used on cold or room temperature food after it has been cooked.
Corn Oil	13.6%	29.0%	57.4%	
Cottonseed Oil	27.1%	18.6%	54.3%	This oil should not be ingested as it contains cyclopropen, which causes toxicity in the liver and inhibits metabolism.
Flax Seed Oil	9.8%	21.1%	69.1%	
Grape Seed Oil	10.0%	16.8%	73.2%	
Hemp Seed Oil	10.0%	12.5%	77.5%	
Palm Oil	51.6%	38.7%	9.7%	
Peanut Oil	18.0%	48.0%	34.0%	
Safflower Oil	6.5%	15.1%	78.4%	
Sesame Oil	14.9%	41.5%	43.6%	

Soy Oil	14.0%	28.0%	58.0%	This is difficult to digest and can be toxic because of this difficulty.
Sunflower Oil	10.8%	20.4%	68.7%	

QUINOA

Now one of my favorite subjects – Quinoa.   I think if I were stranded on an island with only one food I could have with me, it would be quinoa.

- Quinoa is 35 on the Glycemic Index and is the best source of protein for the elderly, the very young, people with diabetes, people with gluten allergies, or anyone and everyone.
- It is the easiest protein to digest because it has never been hybridized.   Since it is so easy to digest, it is the easiest to absorb into the body.   It is the perfect food for the sick, the very young and the elderly, or as stated previously – anyone and everyone.
- Quinoa has more protein than any other grain – an average of 13.8% to 16.2%, compared with 7.5% for rice, 9.9% for millet and 14% for wheat.   Some varieties of quinoa contain 20%.
- Quinoa's protein is a complete protein with all eight essential amino acids with an ideal balance.

- Quinoa's protein is high in lysine, methionine and cystine. It is an excellent food to combine with and boost the protein value of other grains which are low in lysine, or soy which is low in methionine and cystine.
- Besides protein, quinoa provides starch, sugar, oil, fiber, minerals and vitamins and is high in essential linoleic acid.
- It is quick and simple to prepare, taking only 15 minutes to cook.
- Quinoa also contains albumen, which is a protein found in eggs, blood serum and other plant and animal tissues.

Comparisons of the nutritional quality (% dry weight) of quinoa with various grains.

	% dry weight					
Crop	Water	Crude Protein	Fat	Carbohydrates	Fiber	Ash
Quinoa	12.6	13.8	5.0	59.7	4.1	3.4
Barley	9.0	14.7	1.1	67.8	2.0	5.5
Buckwheat	10.7	18.5	4.9	43.5	18.2	4.2
Corn	13.5	8.7	3.9	70.9	1.7	1.2
Millet (Pearl)	11.0	11.9	4.0	68.6	2.0	2.0
Oat	13.5	11.1	4.6	57.6	0.3	2.9
Rice	11.0	7.3	0.4	80.4	0.4	0.5
Rye	13.5	11.5	1.2	69.6	2.6	1.5
Wheat (HRW)	10.9	13.0	1.6	70.0	2.7	1.8

Source for quinoa: Cardoza, A. and M. Tapia. 1979. Valor nutrivia. In: *Quinoa y Kaniwa.* M. Tapia (ed.), Serie Libros y Materiales Educativos No. 49. Reported by J. Risi and H. W. Galwey. 1994. Analyses of the remaining crops reported by: Crampton, E. W. and L.E. Harris. 1969. *Applied Animal Nutrition,* 2nd ed., W. H. Freeman and Co., San Francisco.

Essential amino acid pattern of quinoa compared to wheat, soy, skim milk, and the FAO reference pattern (1973) for evaluating proteins.

Amino Acid	Amino Acid Content (g/100g protein)				
	Quinoa	Wheat	Soy	Skim Milk	FAO
	%				
Isoleucine	4.0	3.8	4.7	5.6	4.0
Leucine	6.8	6.6	7.0	9.8	7.0
Lysine	5.1	2.5	6.3	8.2	5.5
Phenylalanine	4.6	4.5	4.6	4.8	-
Tyrosine	3.8	3.0	3.6	5.0	-
Cystine	2.4	2.2	1.4	0.9	-
Methionine	2.2	1.7	1.4	2.6	-
Threonine	3.7	2.9	3.9	4.6	4.0
Tryptophan	1.2	1.3	1.2	1.3	1.0
Valine	4.8	4.7	4.9	6.9	5.0

Source: Johnson, R. and R. Aguilera. 1980. Processing Varieties of Oilseeds (Lupine and Quinoa), *In: Report to Natural Fibers and Foods Commission of Texas, 1978-1980* (Reported by D. Cusack, 1984, The Ecologist 14:21-31).

Comparisons of the mineral content in quinoa grain with barley, yellow corn, and wheat. Quinoa data are based on the average of 15 cultivars.

Crop	Ca	P	Mg	K	Na	Fe	Cu	Mn	Zn
	%				PPM				
Quinoa	0.19	0.47	0.26	0.87	115	205	67	128	50
Barley	0.08	0.42	0.12	0.56	200	50	8	16	15
Corn	0.07	0.36	0.14	0.39	900	21	-	-	-
Wheat	0.05	0.36	0.16	0.52	900	50	7		14

Source: E. Ballon (1987), personal communication, reported by Johnson (1990).

TONGUE DIAGNOSIS
THE VERY BASICS

The very first rule is, never ever brush or scrape your tongue – the tongue is a diagnostic tool for what is happening at this moment in time in your body. All colors, curdles and whey, are significant, and we need to be able to interpret the signs to use it as a healing tool.

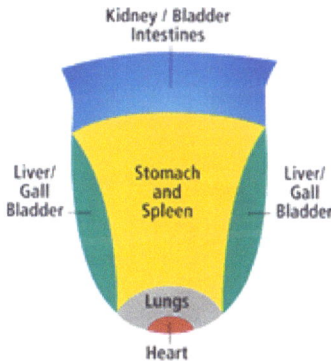

Kidney / Bladder
Intestines

Liver/
Gall
Bladder

Stomach
and
Spleen

Liver/
Gall
Bladder

Lungs

Heart

Here are some very, very, very basic rules for the tongue.   There are whole books written on how to read the tongue, but in general this can give you some information.

- The tongue should be in the shape of a "U". If it is pointed in the shape of a "V", then that indicates heat. If the tongue is doubled up and hard to stick out of the mouth for examination, then it is time to see your Oriental Medicine Physician.
- The tongue should be symmetrical in shape and not deviate to one side.
- The above diagram shows the areas of the tongue that correspond to the organs of the body. For instance, the whole tongue could be pink, but the tip looks really red, it would mean there is heat in the heart area and the other areas would be ok at the time you looked at it.
- The normal color of the tongue is pale red or dark pink. If it is red or purple or pale pink or black or brown or different colors, you need help in diagnosing. The tongue should be all the same color – if there are different colors in different areas of the tongue, that means something is going on in that part of the body indicated on the tongue. Basically if the tongue is red or deep red, dry or cracked there is heat in that area of the body. If it is pale or white there is no blood circulation in that area or you are anemic. If the

tongue is pale or white with lots of saliva, it means internal cold. If the tongue has a white or gray coating it means cold dampness. If it is purple there is stagnation. If there are white or yellow curds on the middle of the tongue, it means you are having digestion problems or you have heat dampness.

- The tongue should be free of holes, cracks, bumps, ridges or cysts.
- The tongue should not have a thick white or yellow coat, or curdy white, yellow, black or brown coating– it should look like it has a little fur on it, but nothing sticky. At the same time the tongue should not be shiny without the fur or have some parts of the tongue missing the fur.
- The tongue should not be oversized – it should be within limits of your teeth. It should not be thick.
- The tongue should be supple and easy to move. It should not be hard and difficult to stick out.
- If the sides of the tongue that correspond to the liver/gallbladder have ridges, it means you are not digesting the food you are eating.
- If your tongue is black or almost white you need to see your physician very soon.
- The tongue should be moist, but not be coated with phlegm.

The tongue changes during the day depending on what we eat and drink, so we can use it to tell how our body reacts to the food, drinks, herbs, vitamins or medications we are taking. By examining the tongue throughout the day it is an indicator as to what we should eat or drink so we can try to bring our body back to normal when we are out of balance.

FACE DIAGNOSIS

In Chinese medicine different parts of the face relate to different parts of the body.

The *FOREHEAD* corresponds to the heart – if your forehead is red or small blood vessels appear as discoloration, it is an indication of either an emotional problem or a heart problem.

The *NOSE* is connected to the stomach, spleen and pancreas network and outbreaks of pimples or discoloration means there is a problem with digestion or constipation. Broken capillaries or redness across the bridge of the nose can indicate heavy stress or alcohol abuse.

The **CHIN** is connected to the kidney, bladder and hormonal system. Dark blemishes around the chin and mouth indicated problems with the kidneys or bladder. Breakouts of acne around the chin and mouth indicate the body has an excess of estrogen, which could affect menstrual cycles and prostate symptoms. If there are blemishes or horizontal lines in the philtrum, the indentation just above your lips, this relates to the uterus or ovaries in women and the prostate in men. In women this could mean a problem such as endometriosis or uterine fibroids.

The **RIGHT CHEEK** relates to the lung and large intestine network. People with a reddish or scaly rash on the right cheek usually have asthma.

The **LEFT CHEEK** relates to the liver and gallbladder network. Broken capillaries or redness indicates high blood pressure and a yellow tongue under the left eye can indicate gallstones or cholesterol.

The **EYES** relate to the liver and gallbladder also. The sclera or white of the eyes should be white – if they are red, it indicates inflammation or strain in the liver and gallbladder area.

pH

So now you know all the information about the types of foods and what they do.   How do we know what it is our body needs?   Well, there are two simple ways – one is to test your pH for acidity or alkalinity, and the other is to learn to read your tongue.   There are many other ways, but these are two of the easiest to learn.   You can purchase pH test strips at any health food store and test your saliva to get a good idea of where your body's pH is at that time.   It is best to test this one hour after you eat or drink something, and that will tell you what that particular food is doing to your body.   It is one of the best learning tools around.   So what does pH do to our body and what is it?

pH is a measurement of acidity or alkalinity in your body after you have eaten food. The pH scale runs from 0-14 with 7 in the middle being neutral. Everything below 7 is "Acid", the lower the number the more acidic; and everything above 7 is "Alkaline". For saliva 7.3 is the ideal body pH.

Each number on the pH scale represents a 10 times the difference from the adjacent numbers. A liquid that has a pH of 6 is ten times more acidic than a liquid that has a pH of 7, and a liquid with a pH of 5 is one hundred times more acidic than 7. For instance, soda has a pH of about 3, making sodas about ten thousand times more acidic than pure water.

When your body's pH is off, it makes it harder for oxygen to get into the cells, mineral assimilation is thrown off balance, enzymes that are helpful become destructive, microbes in the blood can change and become pathogenic, and organs in the body can become compromised and not function 100%. The absorbability of our food, herbs, vitamins and medications is hindered. If our pH is off, we could eat the healthiest food in the world, but our body will not absorb the nutrients in that food. They say that 1000 diseases are a result of an acidic lymphatic system.

The body's pH controls the speed of enzyme activity as well as the speed that electricity moves through your body. In other words, all our biochemical and electrical reactions in our body are controlled by our pH. If we are more alkaline, the electrical energy in our bodies will travel slower with the higher pH.

When the pH is above or below 7.3, enzymes that are normally helpful become destructive, and oxygen delivery to the cells suffers. Research has shown that low oxygen delivery to the cells is a major factor in most degenerative conditions. pH controls the efficiency of insulin, which allows sugar to enter into the cells, which in turn controls blood sugar levels. This is very important for controlling diabetes. Diabetes is called Acidosis, which is too much acid in the body.

When the pH level of the blood is acid, the fatty acids which are normally electromagnetically charged on the negative side, switch to positive and automatically are attracted to and begin to stick to the wall of your arteries, which are electromagnetically charged on the negative side. This is very important for controlling heart attacks and strokes.

Minerals have different pH levels at which they can be assimilated into the body. Minerals on the lower end of the atomic scale can be assimilated in a wider pH range, and minerals higher up on the scale require a narrower pH range in order to be assimilated by the body. For instance, the pH range is wide for sodium and magnesium, narrows a bit for calcium and potassium, and is even more narrow for zinc, copper and iodine. This is why the thyroid can be easily thrown off kilter.

Iodine requires that the pH level is as close to 7.3 as possible in order for the body to assimilate, and it is iodine that is one of the most important minerals needed for the proper functioning of the thyroid. When the thyroid is not functioning properly you have problems with arthritis, heart attacks, diabetes, cancer, depression, fatigue and obesity. Mineral deficiency causes the electricity in our body to slow down tremendously. If we have inadequate mineral absorption in our bodies, we are going to have problems with pH balancing systems.

This is how to balance your pH:

- Follow an Alkaline diet
- Drink Spring Water
- Take a quality magnesium supplement
- Reduce Stress
- Taking Enzymes and minerals along with Green Superfoods with seaweed daily is helpful.
- Reduce acidic foods and liquids.

When the saliva is acidic the following symptoms occur:

- High blood pressure
- Headaches
- Acid reflux (heartburn)
- Acid indigestion
- Hot flashes
- Night sweats
- Heat rashes
- Motion sickness
- Muscle pains
- Insomnia
- Cold feet and hands
- Diabetes

When the saliva is too alkaline, the following conditions occur:

- Bladder infections
- Allergies get worse
- More colds and sinus conditions
- Diarrhea / upset stomachs
- Athlete's foot fungus
- Night sweats
- Itching
- Mold allergies
- Muscle pains
- Headaches

A diet which emphasizes fresh fruit, vegetables and seaweeds, tends to be an alkaline diet.

These foods help when the acidity level is too high (our diet should be 75% alkaline producing):

- All leafy green vegetables and seaweeds
- Whole organic milk (preferably raw)
- Almost all fruits, but not oranges, grapefruit or pineapples.
- Pears
- Papaya
- Bananas
- Soda crackers
- Broccoli (especially raw broccoli)
- Brown rice

- Whole milk yogurt made with cream and active cultures
- Kidney beans
- Higher fat foods,
- Ice cream
- Butter
- Almonds
- Quinoa
- Millet
- Whey
- Most seasonings, but especially cinnamon, curry, ginger and fresh herbs
- Tofu
- Raw vegetables, especially vegetables high in vitamin K
- Chia seeds

When you are too alkaline these foods help (we should only eat 25% acidic foods):
- Probiotic supplements - the bacteria synthesize vitamin K, which help to clot the blood
- Whole milk yogurt with cream on top and active cultures
- Pickles - the acidity helped to balance out the alkalinity
- Corn
- Lentils

- Olives
- Winter squash
- Blueberries
- Cranberries
- Currants
- Plums
- Prunes
- All grains, flours and pastas, other than millet and chia
- All beans and peas, including soy
- Soy milk
- Cheese
- Eggs
- Cashews
- Peanuts
- Pecans
- Walnuts
- All meats, including fish and fowl
- Coffee
- Sugar
- Mustard
- Peper
- Carob
- Vinegar

It is helpful to carry pH strips at all times and test yourself several times a day one hour after you eat or drink to see what it is in your diet that is throwing you off balance. It is a great learning tool.

THE IMPORTANCE OF LYMPHATICS AND HYDRATION

They say that a malfunctioning lymphatic system can cause up to a 1,000 diseases and that it is the basis of our immune system. So what is the lymphatic system? We have our blood system which has large arteries, smaller capillaries, covers our body from head to toe, and is pumped by our heart. The lymphatic system is our water system that covers our entire body and is pumped by the movement of our muscles. By using the pH strips we are testing the acidity / alkalinity of the lymphatic system.

The lymphatics should be in a liquid format, but when we are partially dehydrated, and our electrolytes are not balanced, the liquid turns to gel, which in turn causes lymphatic congestion and toxicity. The lymphatics' job is to eliminate our dead cells that regenerate on a daily basis. It is important to rehydrate using electrolytes, instead of water after heavy exercise.

Living, healthy tissue is always in a state of alignment – proteins die and waste is removed by the lymphatic system. When this waste is not fully removed, we form pathogens and edema, and the cells are not able to get their nutrients. In every serious illness there is a precondition of inflammation resulting in blockage of the lymph nodes where disease begins.

To maintain a healthy lymphatic system, it is important to be hydrated with water and electrolytes. If your lips, eyes, mouth or skin are dry, or if you have dry stools, you are dehydrated. Exercise is the only way the lymphatics can move with the movement of muscles. One of the best exercises is to use a trampoline or rebounder daily.

Lymphatic System

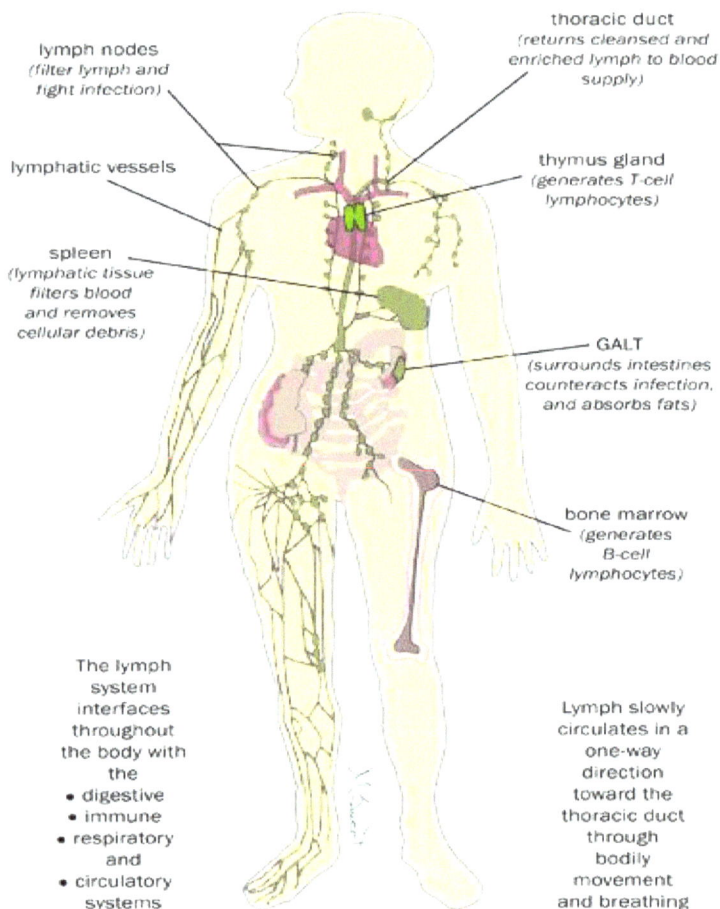

lymph nodes
(filter lymph and
fight infection)

lymphatic vessels

spleen
(lymphatic tissue
filters blood
and removes
cellular debris)

thoracic duct
(returns cleansed and
enriched lymph to blood
supply)

thymus gland
(generates T-cell
lymphocytes)

GALT
(surrounds intestines
counteracts infection,
and absorbs fats)

bone marrow
(generates
B-cell
lymphocytes)

The lymph
system
interfaces
throughout
the body with
the
• digestive
• immune
• respiratory
and
• circulatory
systems

Lymph slowly
circulates in a
one-way
direction
toward the
thoracic duct
through
bodily
movement
and breathing

A FEW NOTES

- Laugh and find humor every day.
- Be thankful for all the family and friends we have in our life daily. If there are problems that arise, try to resolve and forgive them.
- Do not eat food coming out of cans – the cans are made of aluminum and the liners contain a chemical called BHP, which are known carcinogens and contribute to Alzheimer's.
- Avoid nitrates – these are found in lunch meats and other processed foods.
- Drink a good spring water with an alkaline pH and if you use the tap water, filter it to get the chemicals out.
- If you are drinking well water, have it tested at least twice a year to make sure there are no contaminants and heavy metals, and the pH is alkaline.
- Eat fresh organic foods – the more chemicals we can keep out of our body, the better it works.

- Eat in accordance to your body rhythms – since your body's metabolism peaks at around noon time, it is better for your body to have a larger breakfast and lunch and a smaller dinner. If you eat dinner, eat by 6:00 p.m. before the body's metabolism slows down.

- When you sleep, make sure all electronics are off (especially the TV) and the room is dark and quiet. This period of darkness will help to reset your parasympathetic nervous system and will help to reset your body's natural rhythm and health.

- Carry pH strips with you and test under your tongue an hour after you eat to see how your body reacts to the food you just ate. This is one of the easiest biofeedback learning tools around.

- Try to keep your house chemical free to help your immune system.

- Do not cook with aluminum or Teflon coated pots and pans. Aluminum stops the absorption of calcium, causing bone deterioration. Teflon is a known carcinogen. Recent studies show a link of aluminum and breast cancer.

- Take a multivitamin daily – liquid absorbs better than a pill.

- Floss daily – this eliminates plaque build up, which helps with gum and bone disease. Plaque causes chronic inflammation, which increases the chances of heart disease.

- Use a water pick for your teeth and gums daily.
- Stop eating before you are full and eat 3-5 smaller meals a day with the largest meal at noon for the best digestion.
- Exercise daily. Your body needs movement. Exercise your senses – go outside after a fresh rain and breathe in the fresh air, smell the flowers. Dance, golf or play tennis, but do not take the scores seriously – it is just a game. A small trampoline or rebounder is one of the best exercises for use indoors. I have one in front of the TV. Exercise is a great stress reliever. Body movement and brain function are closely related. Muscle movement also moves the lymphatics so you can eliminate the toxins.
- Learn to meditate, pray, chant, hum or sing – take at least 10 minutes a day and be by yourself. If you have children, try to get up at least an hour before they do and center yourself and do the Wake Up exercises.
- Chew everything until it is liquid – remember our stomach does not have teeth, and our body cannot absorb the nutrients until they are in a warm soup

like mixture. The food that our body is able to use equals ENERGY we can use – it is our fuel.

- Beans, nuts, seeds and grains should be soaked in water a couple of hours before cooking so they are easier to digest.
- Don't forget to eat your leafy green vegetables – they are an important source of Magnesium which you need in order to absorb calcium for your bones.
- Do a toxin flush every few months so that it functions better. For one day eat at least five organic apples and drink organic apple juice. Before bedtime drink a mixture of 1/8 cup of extra virgin olive oil along with 3-4 fresh squeezed lemons. In the morning you will see sand or pebbles in your stools. This will help your gallbladder to function better.
- Stay hydrated during the day. If your lips, eyes and stools are dry, you will need electrolytes – best source is unflavored Pedialite or coconut water. Drink spring water, green tea, chamomile tea and other herbal teas. Stay away from soda and alcohol.
- Do not eat or drink anything that says "diet" or "low fat". These products have other chemicals that are harmful to your body.

- Stay away from all GMO products – they are very difficult for you to digest.   Eat organic when possible.
- Try to eat meat only once a week.
- Do not smoke anything – it glues up the lungs so they cannot take in oxygen and shortens your life span.
- If you live near the ocean and it is warm enough to swim – take advantage and swim in the ocean at least twice a week.   If you live near mineral springs take a swim at least twice a week.   If you cannot swim in the ocean or a mineral spring, then take a warm mineral bath at least once or twice a week – your skin is your largest organ and a warm bath takes the toxins out through the skin and it is very relaxing.
- Do not restrict your food – try to eat a wide range of fresh and organic fruits, vegetables, nuts, seeds, and free range meats, chickens and seafood and seaweeds.
- Do not drink while you eat – it dilutes the digestive juices.   Drink one hour after eating or one hour before eating.
- Do not drink cold drinks with ice – better to drink things that are warm or at room temperature.

Your body has to heat everything up when it is ingested, and it will slow your metabolism down.

- Do not use microwaves - Microwave cooking alters food enough to cause, upon ingestion, structural, functional and immunological changes in the body – they transform the amino acid L-proline into D-proline which is a proven toxin to the nervous system, liver and kidneys.

- Do the East West RX Wake Up Exercises first thing in the morning when you wake up to wake up your body and center your energy to start the day. Also take advantage of each time you take a bath or shower to use your towel to massages your whole body and to see if there are sore spots that need to be tapped.

- Don't starve yourself while trying to diet – the body naturally responds by slowing down the metabolism and stores fat. Instead eat smaller meals throughout the day, which will speed up your metabolism.

- Never start the day with cold or raw foods or drinks. These slow down the metabolism. Instead, start the day with warm liquids with lemons and greens to flush out the stagnant foods left in your digestive tract during the night while you slept.

- Use the Glycemic Index on the web which ranks foods according to their effect on blood glucose levels.   Choosing low GI carbs is essential for controlling diabetes and to maintain a healthy weight.   Anything below 55 is a low GI.   A medium GI ranks 56 – 69 and a High GI is 70 and above.   Low GI carbs help you to feel fuller longer, to manage your weight and increases your sensitivity to insulin to improve your blood sugar levels and improve diabetes.

EAST WEST RX WAKE UP EXERCISES

1. Start by sitting upright in a straight back chair with your right foot crossed on top of the left foot. Hold both hands out from the body and then cross your right hand on top of your left hand and clasp them together, at the same time pulling them under so that the thumb of your left hand is touching your chin. Then take several deep breaths through your abdomen. You will feel an energy click between your ears.

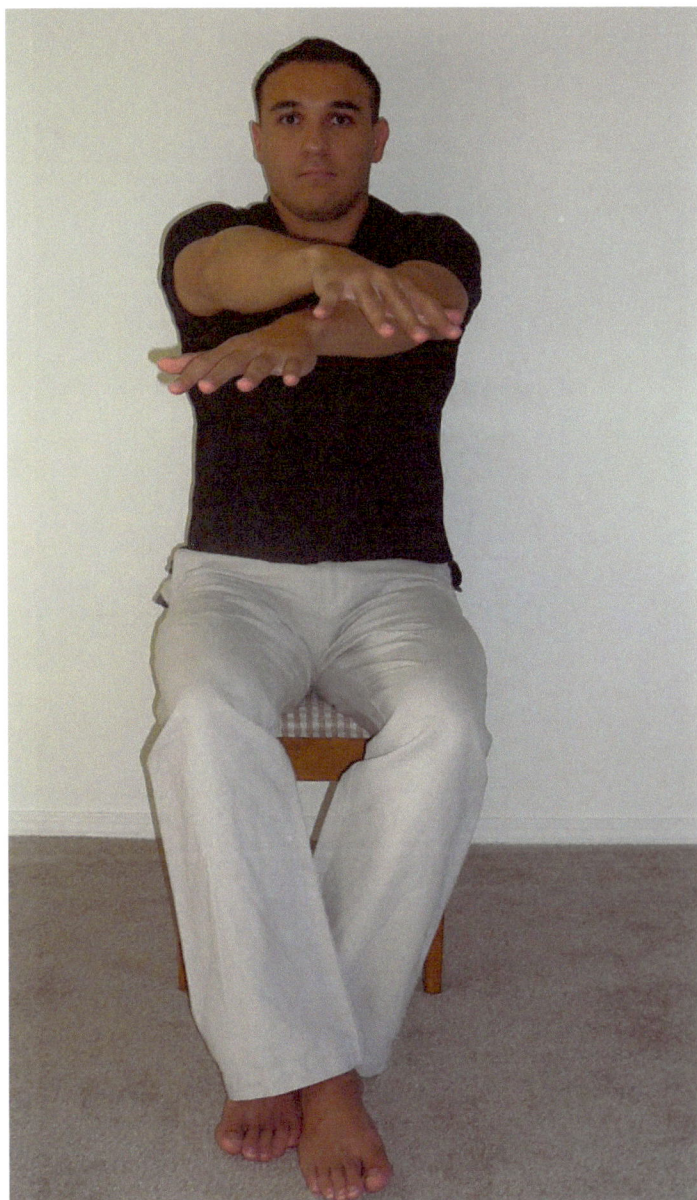

97

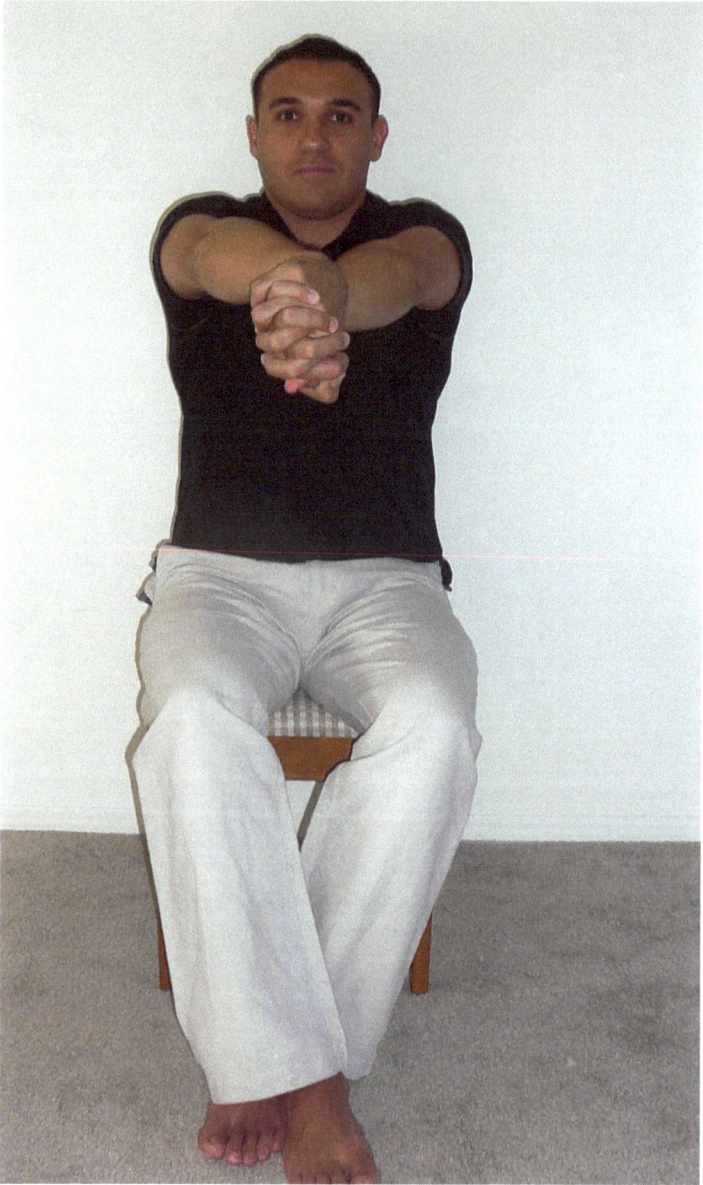

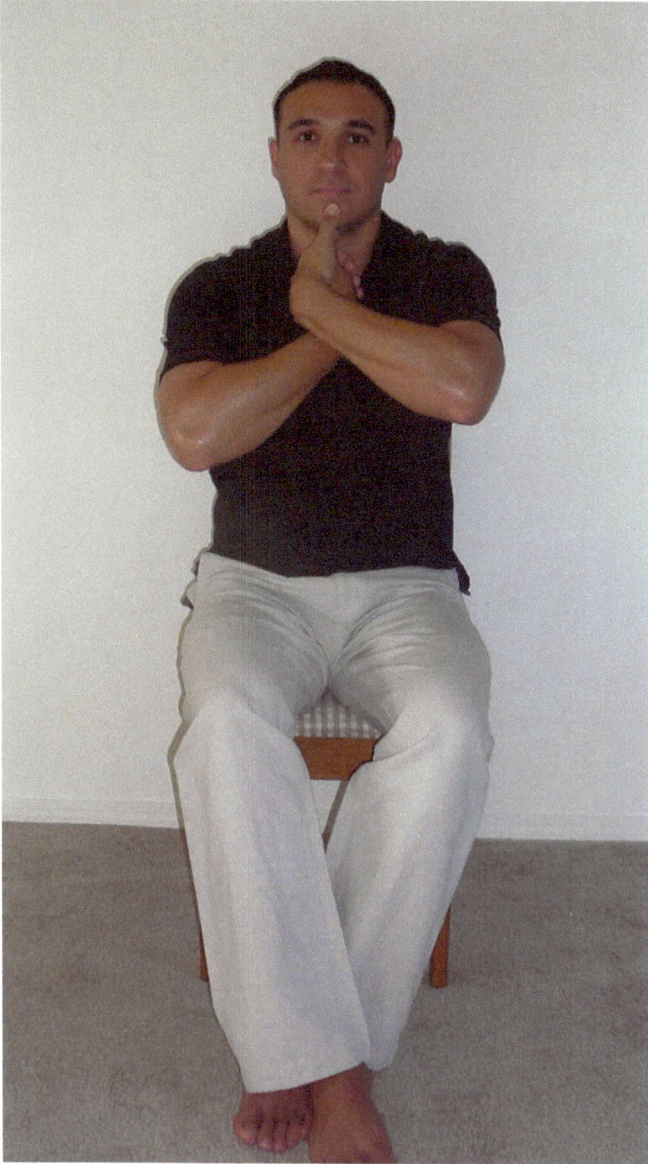

2. Next do the same thing putting your left foot crossed on top of your right foot and repeat as #1. After you take several deep breaths through your abdomen and you feel the energy click between your ears, then unwind and put your feet flat on the ground.

3. Take your left hand and put it flat on your belly button. Take your right hand and clench it like a claw and place it with your finger tips touching surrounding your right ear and breathe through your abdomen several times.

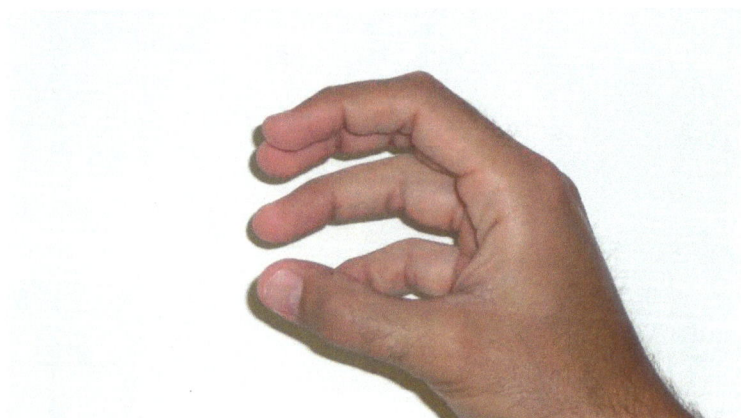

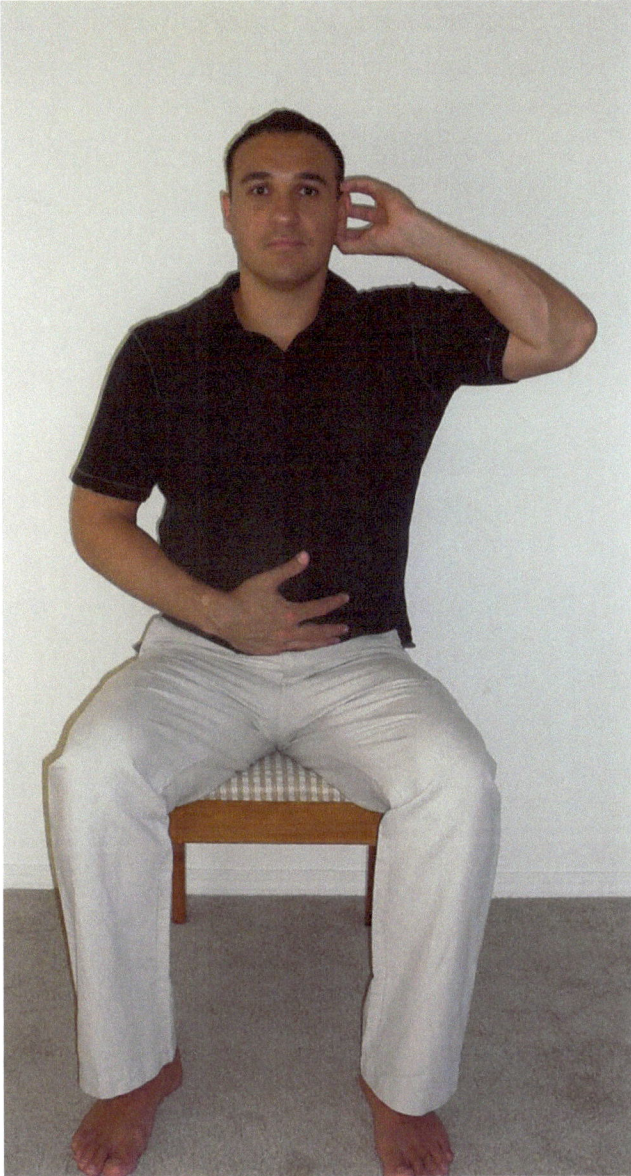

101

4. Keep your left hand on your belly button and take your right hand with your thumb and index finger to rub just below your clavicle several times.

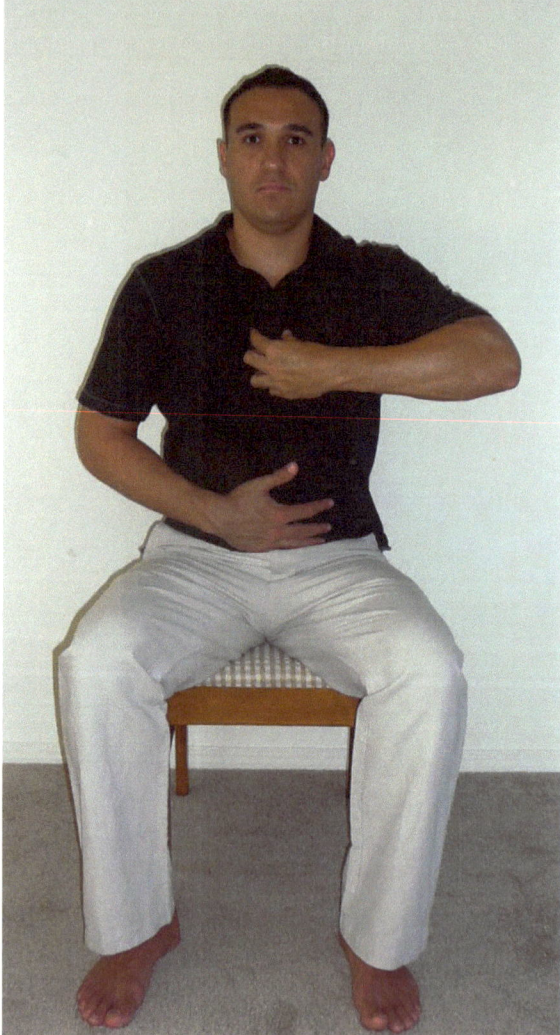

5. Keep your left hand on your belly button and take your right hand with your middle finger and your index finger and place them one on your top lip and one on your bottom lip and rub several times.

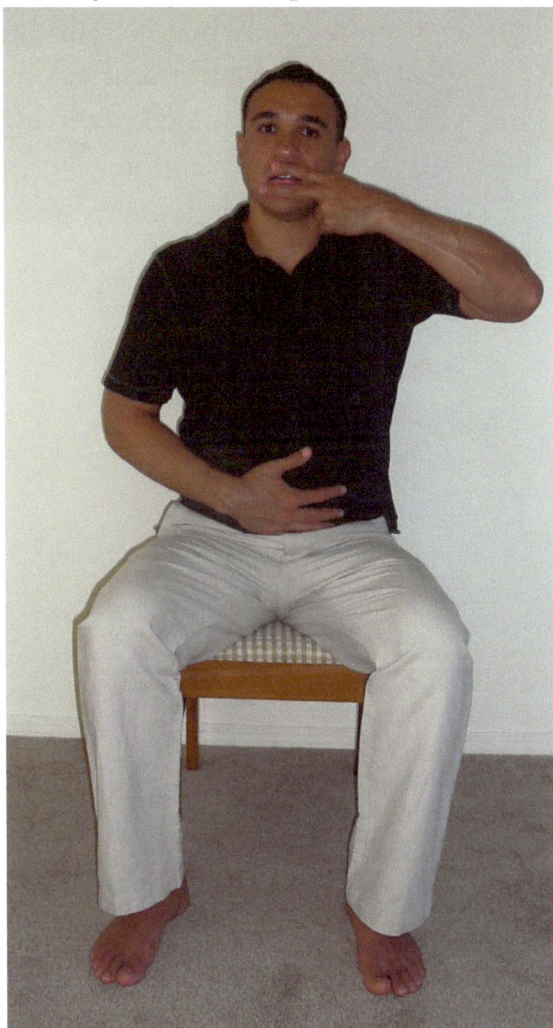

6. Repeat on the opposite side. Take your right hand and put it flat on your belly button. Take your left hand and clench it like a claw and place it with your finger tips touching around your left ear and breathe through your abdomen several times, etc.

7. Take your left hand and put it behind your head and with your right hand take two fingers and put them in your belly button and shake them vertically and then horizontally, and then switch hands.

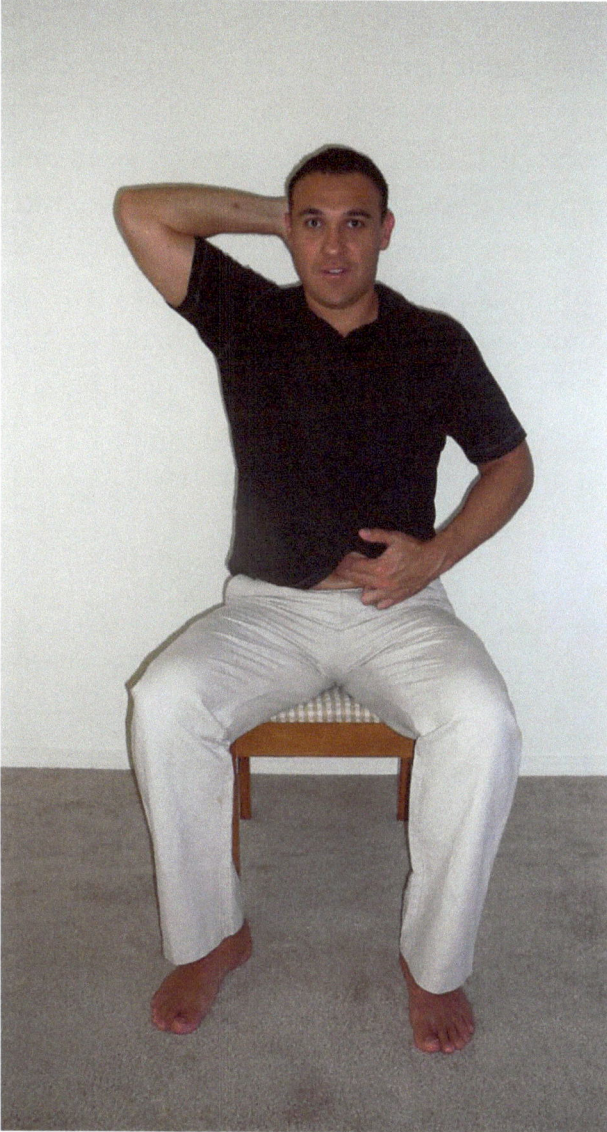

8. Put your left hand behind your head and with your right hand double tap on your head and then on your chest below the clavicle. Keep moving your left hand slowly up the head and keep tapping several times until you reach your forehead. Then switch your left hand to your left ear and double tap your head and then your chest and slowly move your left hand around your head. Then switch with your right hand on your right ear and tap with the left hand slowly moving your right hand around your head.

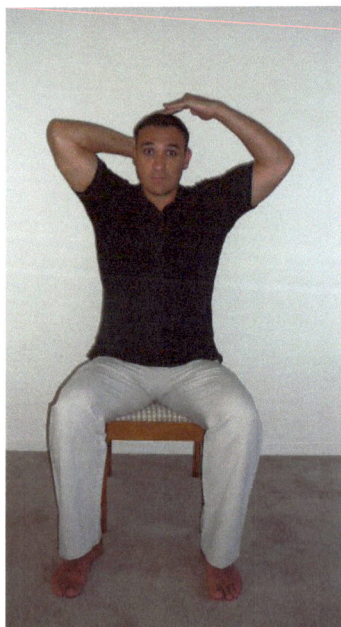

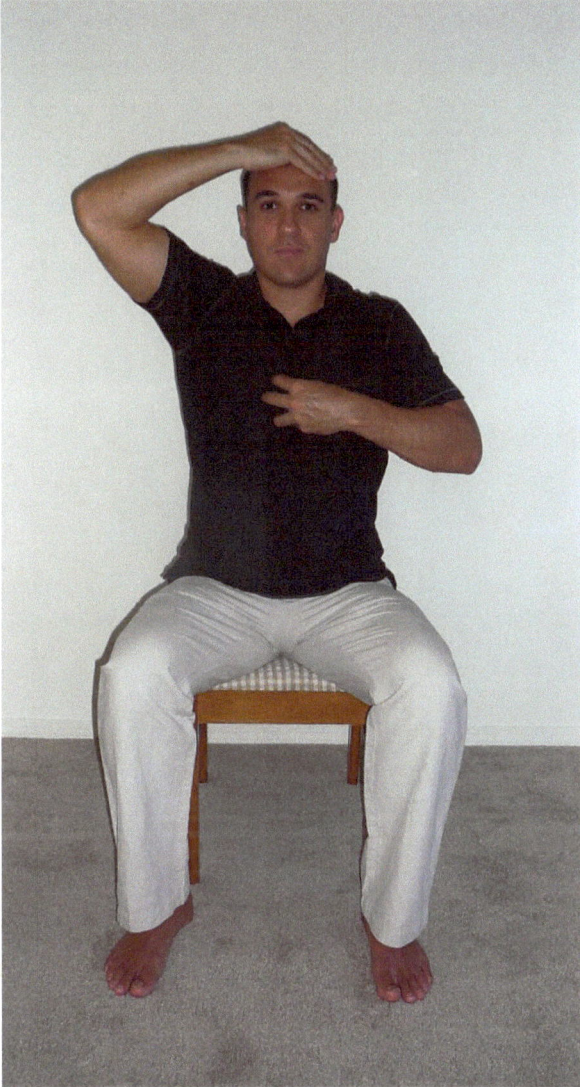

9. Hold your both your ears between your thumb and forefinger and gently massage the ears while gently pulling them outwards starting at the top and go all the way down to the ear lobes.

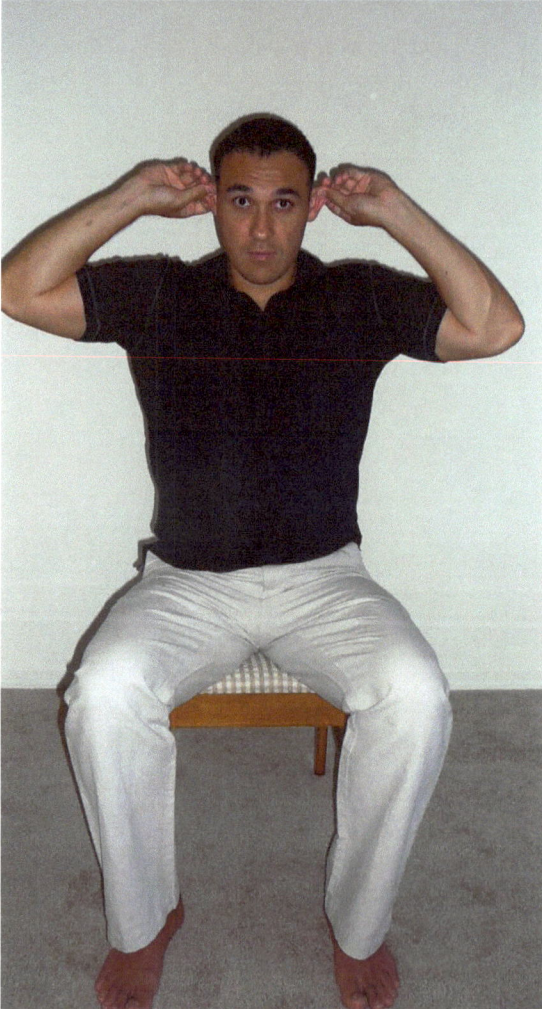

10. With both of your hands in the claw shape tap all over your head and down the back of your neck.

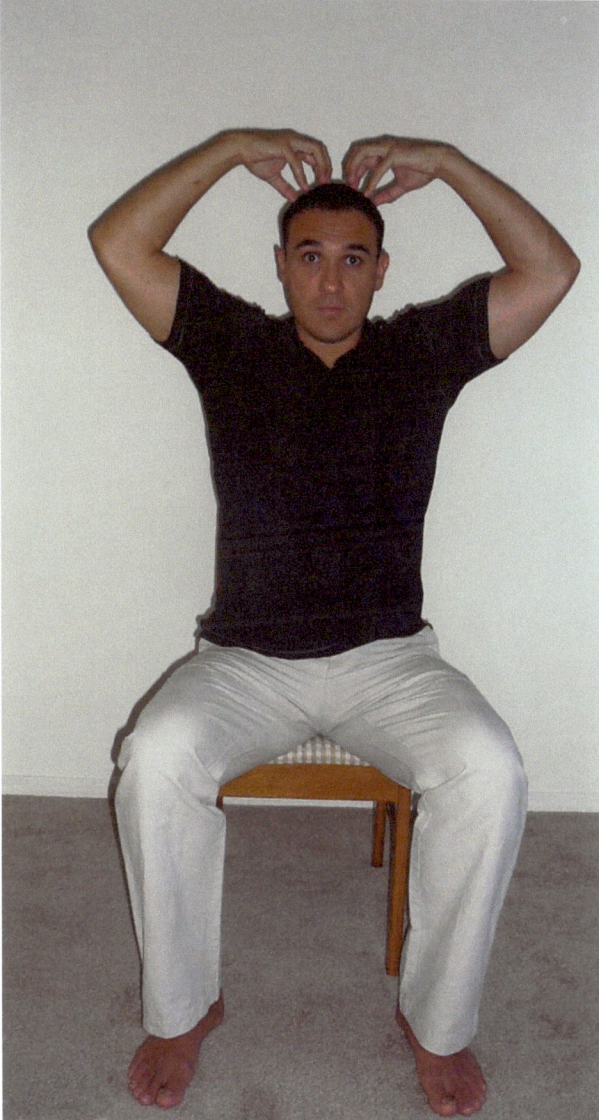

11. Now tap using your opposite hand on your shoulder up to your neck on each side.

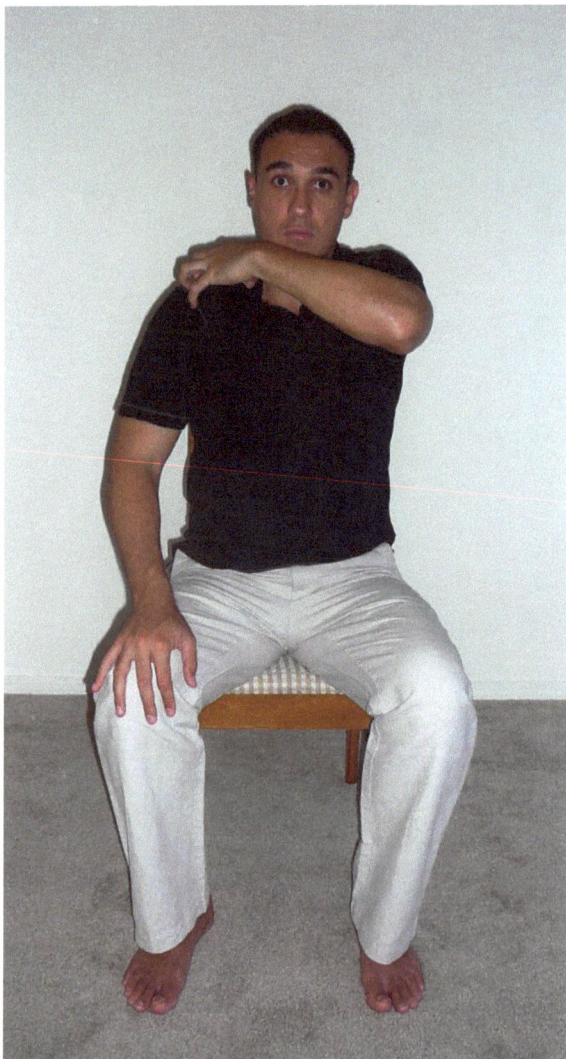

12. Next using your opposite hand tap around your shoulder and your arm pit and follow the arm tapping down to your hands and up again to the shoulder.

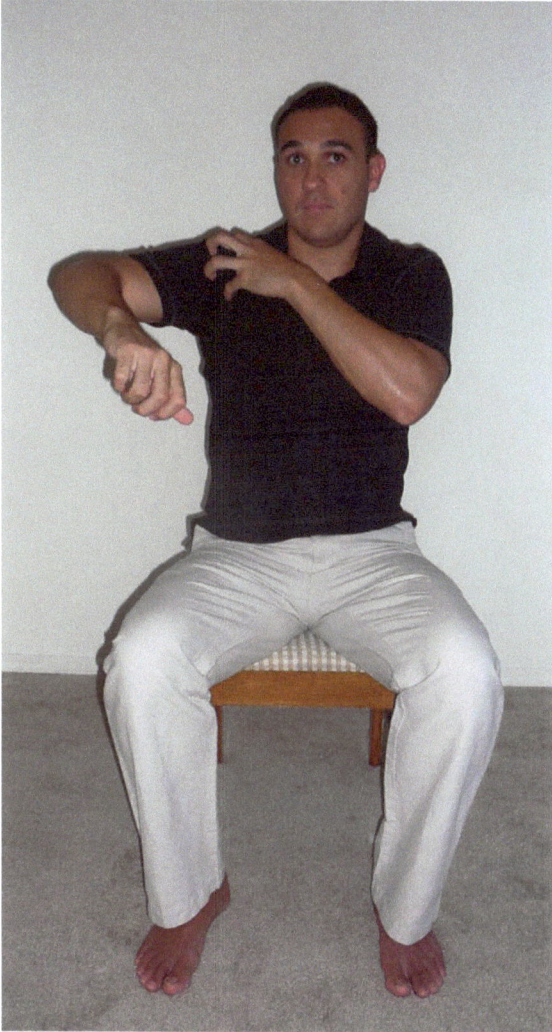

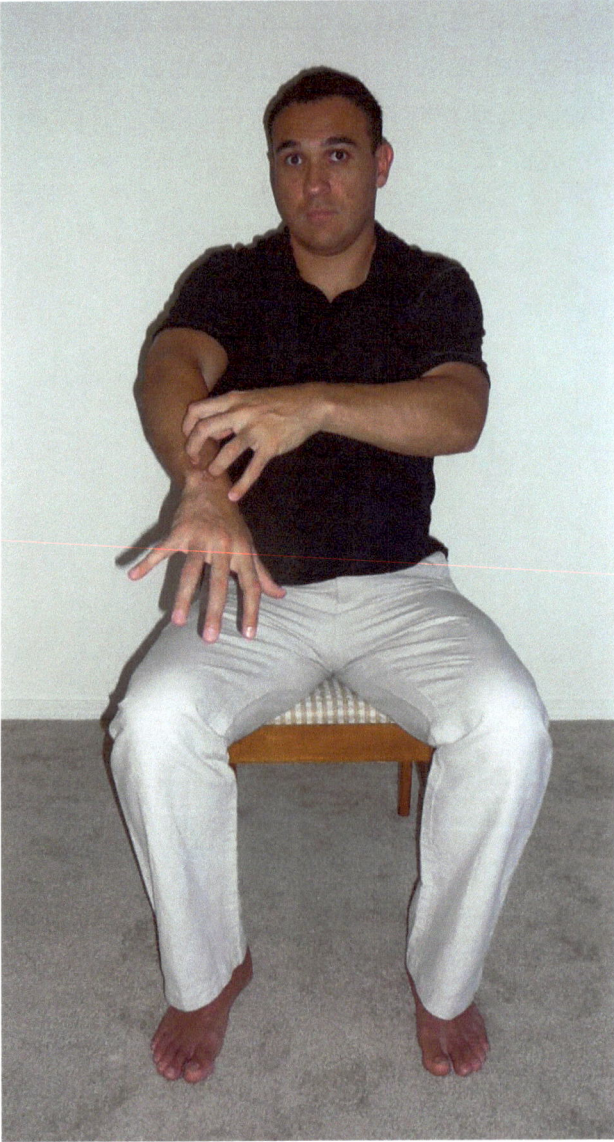

13. With both hands tap the abdomen area going around in a clockwise manner several times.

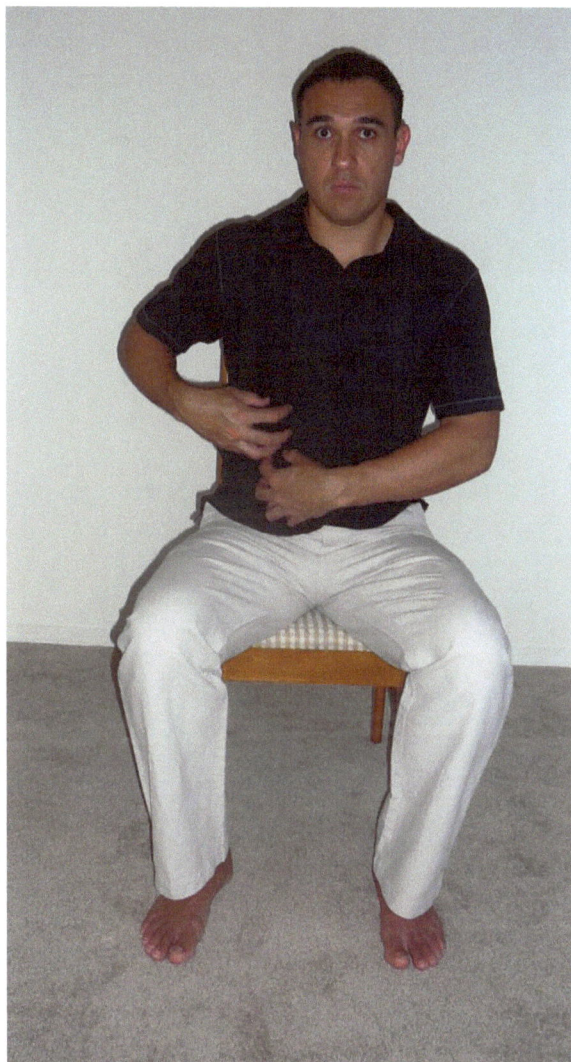

14. Next using your thumbs tap up and down your sides.

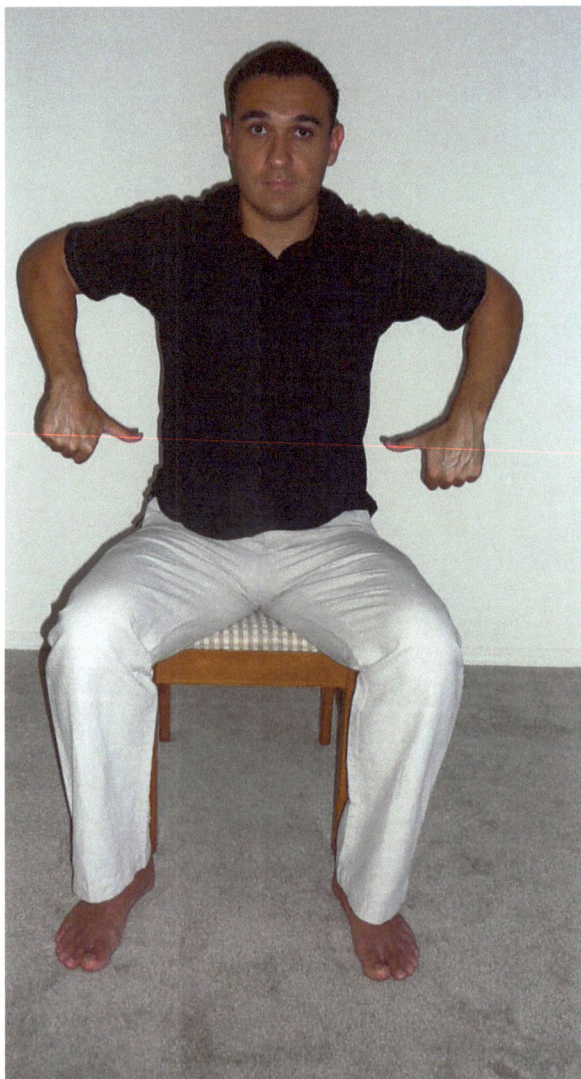

15. Tap your back reaching as much of your back as possible and going down your buttocks and down the outer parts of your legs to your feet. Tap the bottoms of each foot and then tap all the way up on the inner sides of your legs.

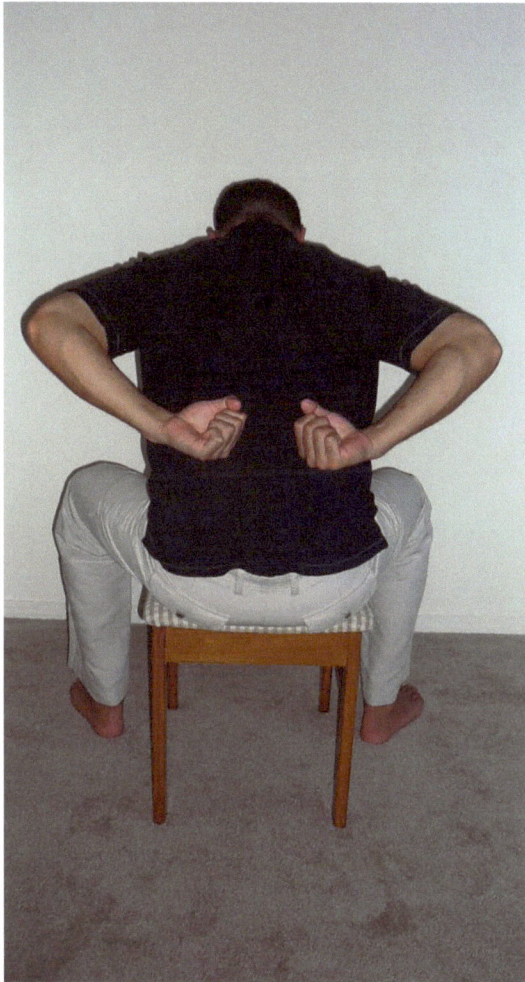

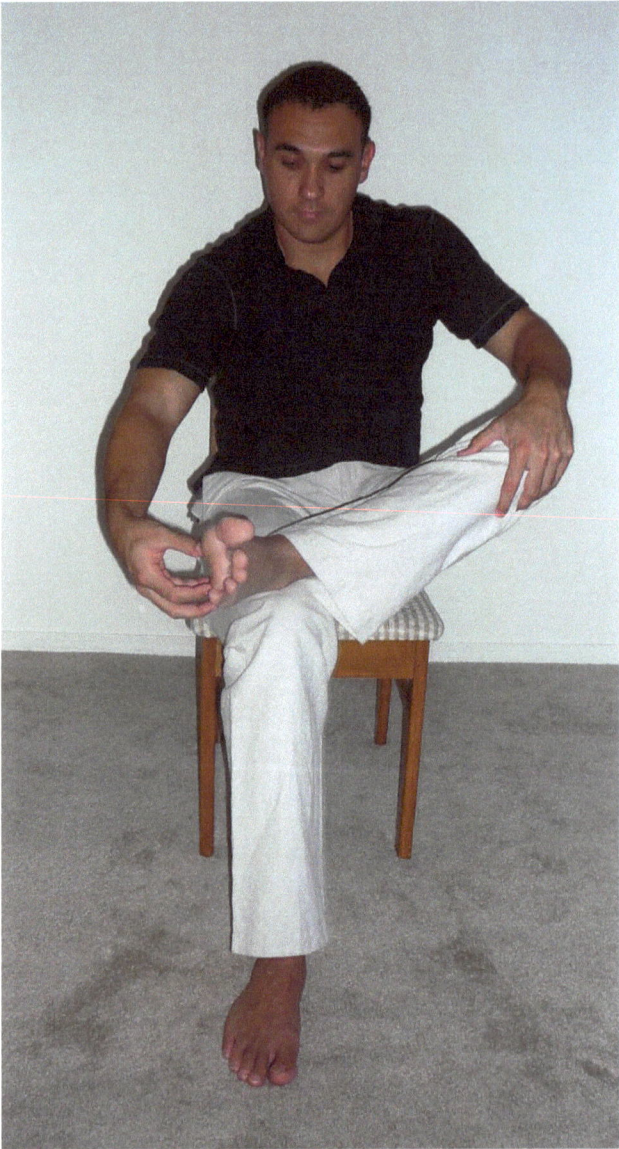

116

16. Tap the back parts of your legs and knees.

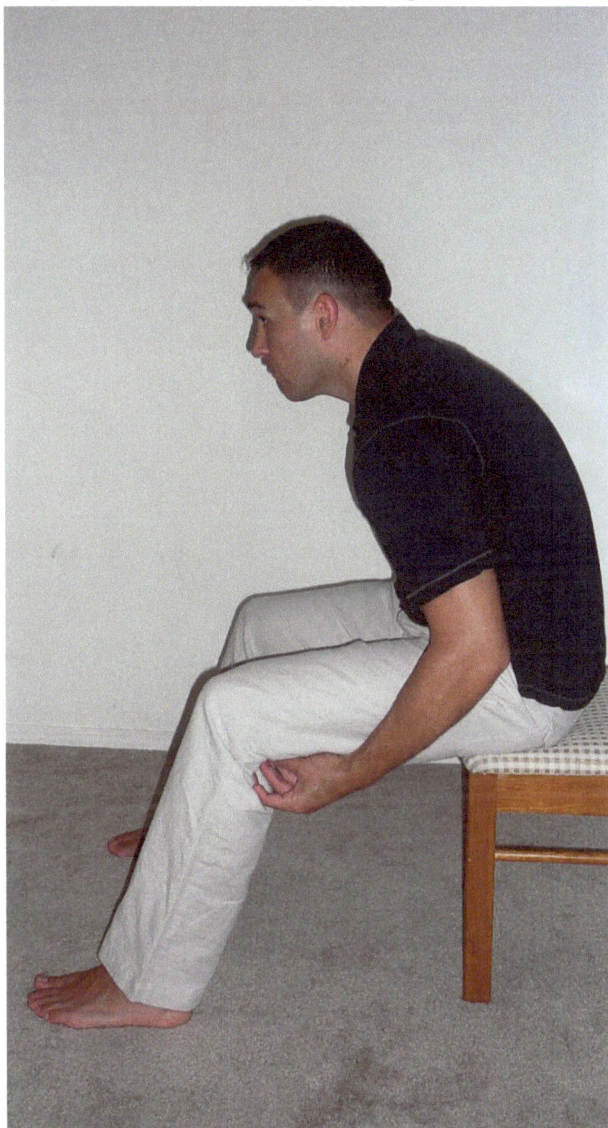

17. Rub both hands together and take each finger on each hand and using your thumb and forefinger rub hard between the area of the finger nails.

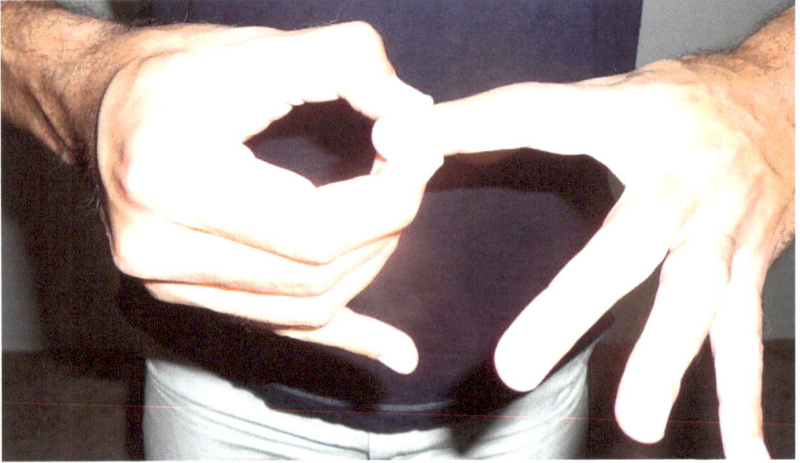

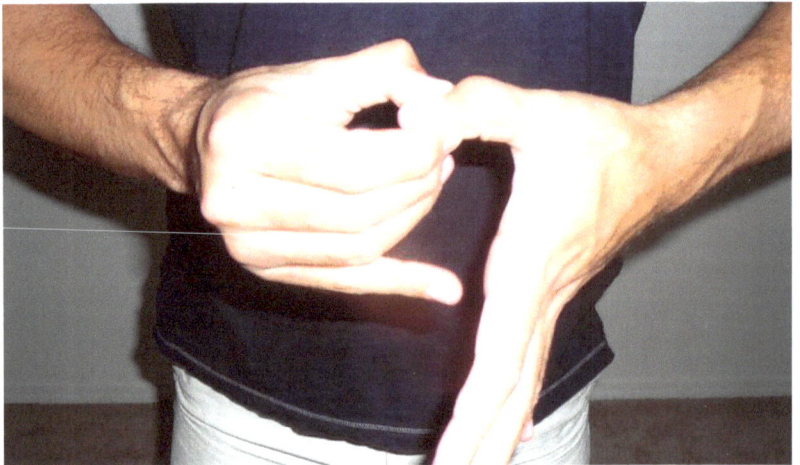

I want to thank my friends, family, and patients who wanted me to write this book. I especially want to thank Ed, Judy, and Jerri, who helped me to put it into a digital format. Thanks to Judy for the donation of the beautiful sky photo on the back cover taken from her back patio.

www.ingramcontent.com/pod-product-compliance
Lightning Source LLC
Chambersburg PA
CBHW040127270326
41927CB00001B/8